THERAPEUTIC MASSAGE AND BODYWORK FOR AUTISM SPECTRUM DISORDERS

VIRGINIA S. COWEN

THERAPEUTIC MASSAGE AND BODYWORK FOR AUTISM SPECTRUM DISORDERS

A Guide for Parents and Caregivers

SINGING DRAGON

London and Philadelphia

First published in 2011
by Singing Dragon
an imprint of Jessica Kingsley Publishers
116 Pentonville Road
London N1 9JB, UK
and
400 Market Street, Suite 400
Philadelphia, PA 19106, USA

www.singingdragon.com

Library of Congress Cataloging in Publication Data
A CIP catalog record for this book is available from the Library of Congress

British Library Cataloguing in Publication Data
A CIP catalogue record for this book is available from the British Library

ISBN 978 1 84819 049 8

Printed and bound in Great Britain
by the MPG Books Group

To Kathleen, Mason, Stephanie,
Ginny, and Pete Jr.

CONTENTS

LIST OF TABLES AND FIGURES

TABLE

FIGURES

ACKNOWLEDGEMENTS

This book has one author, but it was not a truly solo endeavor. It would not have been possible without the help of many people. Thank you to Jessica Kingsley Publishers for recognizing the need to share information on massage for individuals with autism spectrum disorders.

Many thanks to Theresa Crean and Stephanie Hedegard for reading, asking questions, and giving feedback. Thanks to Kate Cowen for your enthusiasm about massage and for this project. Special thanks to Sissy and the children for agreeing to be photographed receiving massage. Thanks to my husband Fred Zlotkin and his children, Felix and Maddie, for their patience with my need for a quiet space to research, write, and edit.

Thank you to my massage students at Queensborough Community College, City University of New York, for contributing to an intellectually stimulating environment to teach and research massage and bodywork. Finally, thanks to all of the parents of children with autism spectrum disorders who have explored using massage. Meeting and working with you and your children has been a wonderful experience.

PREFACE

The idea for this book grew out of many conversations with parents about massage and autism spectrum disorders. In recent years I have had many interesting conversations with parents who were seeking answers to help meet their child's sensory needs. Often they had heard about a specific style of massage, or a nearby practitioner, or they read about the results of a research study. They wanted to know if they should try craniosacral therapy, myofascial release, energy-based massage, or some other style. Sometimes conversations arose from casual meetings. I met people, told them about my career, and they had questions about sensations. They knew their child toe-walked, felt things with the back of the hand, refused to wear certain clothes. They wanted to know why. They wanted to know about massage and bodywork. Specifically how to figure out if a practitioner offered a legitimate therapy or was simply looking to make money. Many parents were interested in trying something new and were curious to know whether massage could and should play a role in their child's sensory therapy. I had to tell them that the answer was not simple. I knew from practice and research that the massage treatment depended on the needs for each individual. I also understood that the expense of daily massages was not practical for many parents who paid out of pocket for other therapies.

Over the years I met many parents who persistently read, asked questions, and sought treatments that would help their child become more aware, engaged, and healthy. Frequently these parents were curious to know why massage was not part of sensory therapy. When they were instructed to brush or stretch their child, they thought massage might offer similar benefits. I knew they were right. Yet I found myself talking less about the benefits or style of massage and more about health policy. Specifically I talked about the limited role of massage in conventional healthcare, legislation governing the practice of massage, and the limitations of health insurance. I found that many parents did not understand how massage practitioners were trained, licensed or certified. They could not figure out who was qualified to massage their child. When they learned that there were options for massage, they were curious. They wanted to know how to locate a practitioner of a style they thought was exotic like Thai massage, reflexology, or even sports massage. Most parents were happy at the possibilities. I met a few parents who were overwhelmed about where to begin. I wanted to help by offering education and suggestions in a non-biased way. Yet I did have a bias. I believed that the most helpful massage practitioners would be trained in the art and science of massage. I also counted on the assumption that the "right" practitioner would put aside expectations and preconceived notions to practice client-centered massage. That meant patiently evaluating how the child might best receive touch, gaining the child's trust, and experimenting with different massage techniques. This was different from typical protocol for a spa or health club massage session.

Along the way I worked with children who had autism spectrum disorders and their parents. All of the children benefited in some way from receiving massage. Many children slept better, some had improved motor skills, and several became more exploratory in their sensory therapy sessions by touching different objects. Frequently the benefits the parents observed were not exactly what would be expected. One child ate entire meals after the massages and tried different foods. Another non-verbal child vocalized more after massage. Yet another would stand facing away from me indicating he wanted back and neck massage. These positive changes were helpful to both the parents and the child. The more I observed them, the more interested I became in reviewing research. I also became a bit confused about why massage was not more often incorporated in treatment.

Since massage is not part of conventional medicine, it is not often recommended by conventional medical care providers who are responsible for healthcare decisions. I have met parents of children with autism spectrum disorders who were told to avoid using any form of complementary or alternative medicine. Their pediatrician, biomedical practitioner, or sensory integration specialist usually lumped massage in with more risky forms of alternative therapies. Sensory therapies were most often received from occupational therapists who are not licensed to massage.

Many parents admitted that they intuitively massaged their child in the hopes of making contact. Some tried to help their child relax and get to sleep. As a practitioner and an educator, I felt it was important to offer parents an explanation of the science of touch, how massage worked, and the potential benefits of different approaches. I understood that enthusiasts for specific massage modalities report that their treatment is *the best.* I also knew that research did not substantiate those claims. The small but growing body of research on massage and issues associated with autism spectrum disorders has found that different types of massage can benefit children with autism spectrum disorders. As a trained massage practitioner and a researcher, I knew that no single treatment approach could be successful to treat a disorder that encompassed a range of individuals with different needs. In practice, this led me to work in an eclectic manner by drawing upon techniques from different modalities. I had an enlightening moment when I found myself performing the same myofascial release techniques on an autistic child who toe-walked and a college basketball player in the same week. Both clients benefited from the treatment and I learned from the experience.

The intention of this book is to provide information for parents of and caregivers for an individual with an autism spectrum disorder. This book does not recommend using massage instead of conventional therapies prescribed by a physician. Rather it aims to help parents and caregivers identify possible therapies that may benefit their child. The book may also be useful to other providers of therapy for children with autism spectrum disorders. It is my hope that by learning and sharing, more children can receive beneficial massage treatments.

1 Introduction

Massage is touch that is systematically applied with the intention to encourage relaxation, relieve aches and pains, promote circulation, and to facilitate a feeling of well-being. While massage is not often a regular part of therapy for a child with autism spectrum disorder (ASD), it offers many potential benefits. There are many different approaches to massage and bodywork from around the world. The words massage and bodywork are sometimes used interchangeably to describe efforts to improve a person's health by touching the body. By definition, massage is a general term used to describe manipulation of the soft tissues of the body that is done for therapeutic purposes. This manipulation can include techniques such as stroking, pressing, kneading, along with joint movements such as stretching. It can also include efforts to manipulate the human energy biofield. Bodywork is a term that is used to describe different types of energy and movement-based styles. Some forms of bodywork include breathing, stretching, and conversation, and are used to engage the client as an active participant in the therapeutic process.

In some areas of the world, massage is routinely used for healthcare. In most Western countries, massage and bodywork are considered complementary or alternative medicine (CAM) because they are not part of the conventional medical system. Surveys in Western countries have found that a large percentage of people use some form of CAM to promote health or treat medical conditions.

In the United States, the National Center for Complementary and Alternative Medicine (NCCAM) recognizes massage and touch-based therapies as a form of CAM. Different styles (also called *modalities*) are grouped into different categories. Styles that focus on muscles and other soft tissues (such as tendons, ligaments, or skin) are considered *manipulative* or *body-based*. These styles rely on information from anatomy and physiology that is used in conventional medicine. Other styles of bodywork that treat the energy of a person's mind/body/spirit are called *biofield therapies*. The existence of an energy field has not been substantiated by scientific research. Yet there are many traditional and newly developed forms of bodywork rooted in the belief that smooth energy flow in and around the body is necessary for good health. Any massage or touch treatment that is taken from a traditional medical system is considered *traditional healing* even when it is used independently of other components of that traditional medical system. NCCAM recognizes that the field of massage and bodywork, along with other forms of alternative medicine, is growing and changing. Globalization has enabled people around the world to learn about and study traditional medicine. Sometimes modern interpretations are fashioned from traditional techniques. Interest and enthusiasm in non-pharmacologic self-care has also contributed to the creation of new forms of massage and bodywork.

The body of research on the benefits of massage has been slowly growing during the past few decades. Studies have evaluated a wide variety of techniques to treat signs and symptoms of many different health disorders including ASD. The variety of massage styles and techniques used in research makes it difficult to draw a single conclusion on the benefits of massage. In general the research results suggest that massage and bodywork do have physical and psychological benefits. Research indicates that massage can increase joint range of motion and decrease physiological measures of stress such as heart rate, blood pressure, and hormones. Massage also promotes relaxation, reduces pain and decreases feelings of depression and anxiety. Studies on massage in infants and children have consistently found that massage can promote healthy weight gain, improve attentiveness, and reduce aggressive behavior and behavior problems.[1-3] A few studies have evaluated the benefits of massage for children with autism spectrum disorders. Findings indicated that massage was helpful in decreasing self-stimulating behaviors, promoting sleep, and increasing receptivity to touch.

Many children with autism spectrum disorders have sensory issues. Occupational therapy aims to help the child manage sensory issues by learning to play, interact socially, manage transitions, and develop fine motor skills. Speech therapy interventions aid in learning to talk and communicate; it can also help with feeding problems. For children with ASD who have poor gross motor skills or too much (hyper) or too little (hypo) muscle tone, stretching and exercise may be learned in physical therapy. Sensory integration therapies are sometimes incorporated into occupational therapy to improve body awareness (proprioception) and balance (vestibular function), encourage appropriate response to stimulation, and assist in development of motor skills. Touch techniques used in sensory integration include tactile play, manipulation of joints, and brushing. This array of therapies is designed to meet the sensory and social needs of each individual child.

For an individual with ASD who has sensory issues, therapeutic massage and bodywork can offer substantial benefits to meet tactile and proprioceptive needs and to address problems with muscle tone. However, it is not routinely used in therapy for ASD. The main providers of therapy for ASD—educators, occupational therapists, and speech therapists—are not trained in massage. Nor are they permitted to administer massage in areas where the massage profession is regulated.

Where regulations exist, they limit the ability to perform massage to licensed or certified practitioners who have substantial training in massage techniques as well as anatomy, physiology, and kinesiology (the study of human movement). Professional massage therapists are trained in the art and science of touch. The art of massage involves listening, feeling, and communicating with the hands, fingers, fists, forearms, elbows, knees, or feet. The science of massage is based on training in anatomy and physiology of the human body including extensive study of the muscles, bones, joints, nerves, and circulation.

The art and science of massage intersect when the massage practitioner chooses appropriate techniques, and alters or adjusts the techniques based on feedback from the client. This feedback may be verbal, but more often it is visual or tactile. Visual feedback is gleaned through observed changes in facial expressions, breathing patterns, or body positions. Tactile feedback is felt through changes in the pliability or temperature of skin and muscles and the relaxation or increase of muscle tension. Many massage therapists are trained in different styles of massage. Regardless of the particular style or techniques used, massage therapists are taught to communicate through touch.

Despite popular claims, no single type of massage therapy is known to be better than another for ASD. The different sensory issues presented and the possibility for massage to address these issues varies considerably among individual children across the autism spectrum. A single massage style is not likely to successfully meet such a wide variety of needs. The success of massage for ASD relies on using appropriate techniques that are selected based on each child's unique sensory integration difficulties. For one child that might mean a gentle craniosacral therapy session, while another might respond best to a vigorous Swedish massage. Still another child might need a more eclectic approach that draws from a massage style that has a broad array of techniques or a treatment that integrates aspects of massage from several different styles. A parent or caregiver has many choices ranging from an eclectic practitioner who is experienced at practicing different styles of massage to seeking treatment from many different practitioners who are each experts in a single style. What is important is to match the intervention to the sensory needs of the individual with ASD.

The term *pediatric massage* refers to any type of massage given to infants and children. It can refer to general massage performed by a massage therapist. A unique aspect of pediatric massage is teaching parents to massage their children. For a typical child, this is often recommended to help the child sleep or to encourage bonding between the parent and child.

The sensory stimulation of massage can increase or decrease arousal of the nervous system. For a typical massage client, pressure and strokes are considered to be either stimulating or relaxing. Deep pressure, compression, kneading, and stretching techniques are stimulating techniques. Light pressure, gentle rubbing, and slow range-of-motion techniques are relaxing techniques. Selection of the appropriate techniques in massage for each massage client can promote a desired effect on the nervous system. In children with ASD, the choice of stimulating or relaxing strokes is more complicated. With sensory problems, the response to a stimulus is often unpredictable. Sometimes deep pressure can be more relaxing than light pressure, whereas light pressure may be more stimulating. Knowledge of how the body perceives touch can help make this a more logical and beneficial process.

The myriad of massage and bodywork options available can be confusing. Yet, the opportunity for choice offers a lot of hope for parents seeking a touch intervention to supplement their child's therapies. What is most important is to attempt to find the style of massage or bodywork that can help to treat a child's tactile problems and complement their other therapies and treatments.

HOW TO USE THIS BOOK

This book provides an overview of massage and touch and addresses how massage and bodywork can benefit a child with ASD. It is not intended to be a "how to" guide. Rather it provides information to help parents and caregivers make choices that are best for their child's care. Everyone has a preference for how he or she prefers to be touched. But parents' preferences may not be shared by their child. This is especially true for a child with ASD who has sensory problems. That is an important consideration because preference for touch is an essential factor in encouraging receptivity to touch. The book's emphasis on massage and bodywork focuses specifically on the touch-oriented or sensory benefits for a client with ASD. This book may also be useful for any clients with sensory problems, as well as proprioceptive or motor skill difficulties.

The aim of this book is to help parents and caregivers understand the variety of massage and bodywork styles as well as understand how to choose a style that has potential as an addition to the therapy program for their child. For readers who have received professional massage, some of the styles discussed herein may be familiar. Others might be less well known because the field of massage and bodywork is very broad. Sometimes the unknown can hold the key for a client with ASD. If parents have a basic awareness of other styles, they may be more open to pursuing massage and bodywork for their child. It might be necessary to find a practitioner who takes an eclectic approach to treatment or to visit several practitioners who specialize in one style in order to find the right therapy for a client with ASD.

The terminology used in this book has been selected to be inclusive, compassionate, and instructive to the reader. The terms *parents* and *caregivers* are intended to be inclusive referring to any adult who has a responsibility caring for a child with ASD. Sometimes the caregiver may not be the biological parent of the child. When only the word parent is used in context, it does not exclude non-biological caregivers for the child. It is used for readability. The author assumes that any reader of this book (regardless of the relationship) has a caring interest in how massage can help someone with ASD.

Therapeutic massage and bodywork in the various forms offer potential benefit to anyone of any age. This book refers to the *individual with ASD* to encompass any individual with an autism spectrum disorder. This acknowledges the treatment needs and potential benefits of massage for adolescents and adults with ASD as well as infants and children. The word *typical* is used in reference to anyone who does not have an autism spectrum disorder.

In general, the words patient and client are both used to describe the receiver of massage. Because massage is not part of conventional medicine in Western countries, the term patient is sometimes viewed as misleading. Massage is also most often performed outside of the medical setting. To be inclusive of the possible applications, the massage recipient will be referred to as the *client*.

Various titles used by professional massage practitioners include: massage therapist, masseuse, therapeutic bodyworker, and movement educator. In some areas of the world, where massage is part of the traditional medical system, the massage practitioner may be called doctor. There is substantial variety in the rules that regulate professional massage practices and who is eligible to give massage treatments in the United States, the United Kingdom, and Canada. Owing to the many possible titles for the giver of massage, the word *practitioner* will be used to describe the person giving the massage treatment.

The book is organized into three parts. The first part of the book, "Understanding Massage and Sensation," provides information about massage, the sense of touch, and how massage and bodywork may benefit patients with ASD. This can aid parents and caregivers to understand why a child with ASD may have problems with touch, sensation, or proprioception, and how this fits with the characteristic signs presented by the child. The second part of the book, "Exploring Styles of Massage and Bodywork," describes specific types of massage (modalities). For each modality the history, theory, and techniques are presented. Where available, general research on a modality or on how the modality may impact ASD is reported. The modalities are grouped into three categories: anatomy-oriented massage, energy-based bodywork, and other styles of therapeutic bodywork. The final part of the book, "Trying Massage for Your Child," offers recommendations on how to select a style of massage and locate a practitioner. It also gives general precautions, tips on preparing the client for massage, and suggestions for working with the massage practitioner. Asking the right questions, creating a nurturing environment for a child to receive touch, and experimenting with different types of massage can help increase the success of massage as an additional therapy.

This book will help you to educate yourself about the possibilities for massage as a complementary therapy. Remember that what you enjoy in massage may not be enjoyed by your child. You might even learn about a modality that sounds interesting for you to try for your own health and well-being. Taking a first step by reading this book can open the door for you and your child to the benefits that can be received from the wonderful world of therapeutic massage and bodywork.

PART 1

UNDERSTANDING MASSAGE AND SENSATION

2 Massage and Bodywork

Therapeutic massage and bodywork are the application of touch or manipulation to improve health and well-being. Massage is used for health-related reasons, but it is not often considered conventional healthcare. It is a natural or holistic approach that has a lengthy history around the world. There are many different interpretations used in massage and bodywork. While touch is used for nurturing and communication, massage and bodywork are different. They involve deliberate use of techniques. The benefits of massage are related to the techniques used in massage treatment.

DEFINING MASSAGE

Massage does not have a single beginning or point of origin. It has a long history in Europe, Asia, and in other places around the world. The word *massage* is a combination of Greek and French words for *kneading* and *pressing*. In Ancient Greece, passive and active movements were used as a form of exercise. Vigorous rubdowns were provided in Italy and Turkey in bath houses. The earliest writings about massage as a therapy can be traced to China and "The Yellow Emperor's Classic of Medicine." Pressure, stretching, and massage were used as part of holistic healing. As a medical therapy, it has a long tradition elsewhere in Asia including Thailand and Japan. There is also evidence that massage techniques were practiced in the Middle East in Persia and Egypt. Massage has an extensive tradition as a healing art.

Massage in its various forms is considered to be complementary or alternative medicine because it is not part of the current conventional, biomedical system in the United States, Canada, the United Kingdom, and Australia. Complementary and alternative medical treatments are covered by the acronym CAM. Other healing arts that are considered to be CAM include: chiropractic, naturopathy, ayurveda, yoga, and acupuncture, as well as vitamin and herbal supplementation. The classification as CAM does not necessarily mean that these therapies are less effective than conventional approaches. They are just an alternative.

It is important for parents to understand the difference between using massage as a complementary therapy or as an alternative to conventional medicine. Massage is not a substitute for any other therapy prescribed by a physician, but massage is used as a therapeutic intervention for ASD. The aim of massage is to support or enhance the conventional treatment. For an individual with ASD, this means that massage would complement a biomedical stimulant used to increase physiological arousal. When massage is used instead of another therapy, it is considered alternative. The substitution of massage would aim to produce the same outcome as the other therapy. In this way, massage would be an alternative to the brushing treatment used in sensory integration therapy.

Western or European styles of massage are based on conventional medical anatomy and physiology of the body. This anatomy and physiology was learned by dissecting the body to understand how it works. In Western styles of massage, techniques are systematically applied to muscles and connective tissues (ligaments, tendons, joint capsules, skin, and fascia) to relax tension and improve circulation. This approach to massage is closely related to conventional medicine because it is based on the same understanding of the body.

Massage styles that come from Asia, India, and other Eastern countries are often referred to as *bodywork*. The treatment may include massage techniques along with pressure, stretches, exercises, and manipulations. Many Eastern modalities have approaches that are not based on anatomy but are rooted in traditional medical systems or "folk" medicine. These traditional systems are holistic, intending to treat the patient's mind and spirit as well as the physical body. This type of medical system is based on observations of the natural environment, how the patient interacts with the environment, and universal energy. Within these medical systems, massage is often an important part of healthcare. It may be used alongside herbal medicines, nutrition, bathing, exercise, and meditation. The goal of medical care and massage is to maintain a balance of the patient's energy.

The term "bodywork" is also used to describe an array of hands-on therapies that aim to improve posture, increase joint range of motion, increase self-awareness, or promote overall well-being. Some of these therapies have ancient origins while others are modern interpretations of traditional concepts. Many forms of bodywork have emerged throughout the world in recent years. These styles are sometimes based on a combination of anatomy and energy. Sometimes they are interpretations of portions of traditional medical systems. They may take a psychosocial approach by including verbal cues and feedback. Overall the goal of the treatment is to restore balance to the patient's mind and body. What they have in common with massage is that they are somatic therapies. A somatic therapy is an approach that treats the muscles, bones, or nerves and can also have an effect on a person's psychological well-being. In this way, somatic therapies' purpose is to holistically treat a person in order to improve their health.

BENEFITS OF MASSAGE

Massage can promote circulation, reduce inflammation, increase joint range of motion, and help alleviate muscle soreness. Most people agree that massage feels good. It can be relaxing or invigorating depending on the techniques used. Slow, gentle strokes help to calm and relax; brisk strokes are invigorating. A professional massage therapist selects specific massage techniques to treat the needs of the client. These needs are identified through a process called assessment. A pre-massage assessment can include interviewing the client about health history and activities, observing the client's movements or posture, and conducting tests that evaluate the range of motion of joints and muscles.

Researchers have studied the effects of massage on disorders and diseases. A wide variety of massage styles and session lengths have been evaluated in research to date. The good news is that massages which last anywhere from ten to ninety minutes, or even two hours, can benefit the client. More good news is that research has identified benefits from different styles of massage. The bad news is that the field of massage research is not very big and the components that are included in massage can vary tremendously. The challenges that are involved in drawing research conclusions in general do not mean that massage lacks benefit. Rather it points toward the adaptability of massage and bodywork in treating symptoms related to a variety of physical, emotional, and psychological conditions. One challenge in evaluating massage is that it is difficult to design a standardized treatment for research. Massage therapists are trained in evaluation and treatment design. That means they select techniques that they believe will provide the most benefit to their client—at that moment in time—based on the client's needs and expectations. This is called *client-centered* massage. The approach is flexible and prescriptive rather than a strict, predetermined, automatic sequence. For example, consider massage for a client who suffers from tension headaches compared to a client who is recovering from a knee injury. With the "headache" client, the massage therapist would spend more time focusing on the neck, upper back, chest, head, and arms. The session goal would be to relax muscle tension in this area. With the "knee injury" client, the massage therapist would spend more time on the hips, legs, and maybe even the low back. The session goal would be to reduce any inflammation in the knee, lower leg, and foot (on the injured side) and release tension in muscles that might be sore because the client altered his gait to accommodate the injured leg. If both clients schedule a one-hour, full-body massage, the amount of time devoted to the various areas of the body would be different. The techniques used on the focused areas would be different even though the session was the same length. This means the actual client-centered massages would be different for each person. Massage therapists also may change the techniques used in treatment for the same client who is seen for multiple massage sessions. Again, the selection of techniques is based on assessment of the client's condition which can change over time.

Massage for an individual with ASD must be client centered. Careful assessment is the key to understanding the client's needs. Massage can be used to meet sensory needs, breakdown tactile defensiveness barriers, and reduce muscle tightness. It also can be used to help the client understand the concepts of discernment, proprioception, and communication through touch.

SENSORY PROCESSING AND MASSAGE

Somato-sensory problems are common in individuals with ASD. *Somatic* means body and *sensory* refers to the sensitivity to stimuli from the surroundings. Somato-sensory problems include difficulty feeling, moving, and understanding the physical body. For a typical child, movement ability (*motor skill*) is developed with practice. The integration between nerves and muscles parallels the child's growth. Sports-based skills like kicking or throwing a ball, running, and jumping are *gross motor skills* that help develop coordination, balance (*vestibular function*), and awareness of the position of the body (*proprioception*). Eating with utensils, coloring, or writing with a pencil are *fine motor skills*. These skills require a more precise type of coordination that improves with practice. The ability to execute gross and fine motor skills through movement depends on the ability to understand the task along with the integration of different body systems including the nervous, muscular, skeletal, skin, and endocrine systems. For reasons that are not clearly understood, children with ASD often have poor motor skills, lack proprioceptive awareness, or have vestibular problems. This can be accompanied by a problem with muscle tone and sensory issues.

When an individual with ASD has somato-sensory problems, it is called *sensory integration dysfunction* or *sensory processing disorder*. This is characterized by motor skill difficulties, trouble with awareness of the position of the body, and sensitivity to stimuli. Often the individual with ASD displays inappropriate reactions to stimuli which is shown by ignoring or over-reacting to certain types of stimuli. Someone with sensory processing problems may be insensitive or overly sensitive to sights, sounds, tastes, smells, or touch. Closing the eyes, covering the ears, pinching the nose, and closing the mouth are often coping behaviors. These are ways to censor information by limiting stimulation from bright lights, loud noises, strong smells, unpleasant tastes, or undesirable textures. Sensitivities to touch and physical contact can involve extreme sensitivity or lack of sensitivity to stimuli. Because most of the body is involved in receiving and comprehending touch through stimulation, it can be a difficult sense to understand. It is very hard to filter the awareness of touch. Sensory integration problems can lead to tantrums or withdrawal when individuals with ASD have trouble understanding, navigating, or communicating within their surroundings.

Individuals with ASD are often broadly classified as hyper-sensitive or hypo-sensitive to touch. Some may be a combination of both, depending on the area of their body that is being touched. When individuals with sensory processing problems exhibit unusual sensitivity to touch, it may be reflected in only the hands or feet. It may also be relevant to different types of physical contact on other areas of the body.

An individual with ASD who is generally *hyper*-sensitive to touch might be extremely ticklish, as well as resistant to bathing, grooming, and diaper changes. Because the hands and feet have many sensory receptors, hyper-sensitive individuals often walk on their toes and touch things with the back of the hand rather than the palms and fingers. They are trying to limit the contact of their sensitive hands and feet with the ground or objects as a way to filter stimuli. Their subconscious is trying to limit the sensory information that their brain must process. When they encounter lights, sounds, smells, or tastes that are overwhelming, it is fairly easy to remove the stimulus. But it is harder with touch, so they are creative in filtering the stimulus. A hyper-sensitive individual would likely be most receptive to massage that uses light to moderate pressure and gentle movements. For this individual, using the same massage sequence repeatedly would be important so that the session became familiar and predictable. It may take a long time for hyper-sensitive individuals to be receptive to touch on the hands or feet.

An individual with ASD who is under-responsive to touch is called *hypo*-sensitive. This individual may be unaware of light touch, may not respond to tickling, and not be bothered by minor injuries like cuts and bruises. Hypo-sensitive individuals may also hit, kick, bite others or bang their own head. This may be done to communicate—especially for someone who is not verbal. They may be trying to gather information about their environment. It is also possible that self-injurious behavior takes place because the individual has problems discerning through touch. They may have trouble understanding the boundaries of their own body. Hypo-sensitive individuals with ASD would likely be receptive to deep pressure, rubbing, or kneading. This person may not be receptive to massage at first because they have problems feeling. Joint range of motion, stretching, and muscle compression would help to promote proprioceptive awareness.

The differing styles of massage and bodywork offer a vast menu of touch therapies to choose from for the various sensitivities that are apparent across the ASD spectrum. A general understanding of massage can help illustrate possible applications of massage for ASD. Massage techniques like range-of-motion, stretching, and compression are routinely used in modalities like sports massage, myofascial release, and neuromuscular massage to promote proprioceptive awareness. It is believed that passive movement applied to athletes who are relaxed can help athletes understand the position of their body on a subconscious level. Massage and passive movement are also used in rehabilitation for injuries. Any stimulation of muscles or joints through massage or movement activates the sensory receptors of the nervous system on some level. Whether this stimulation creates an arousal of the nervous system on a conscious level or subconscious level, it can be beneficial. For the same reasons that massage and movement can benefit athletes or injury rehabilitation, it can also benefit symptoms in an individual with ASD who has sensory or motor problems.

For both fine and gross motor skill problems, massage can be beneficial in stimulating muscles that are needed for both motor movements. Lack of muscle tone would impede the individual's ability to develop muscle strength and coordination. Excessive tightness in muscles and fascia is characteristic of too much muscle tone. This can cause problems with either fine or gross motor skills. Massage can be used to stimulate muscles and promote circulation. It can also decrease tension in habitually tight muscles which can— inversely—be helpful to the muscles lacking tone or strength.

Research on massage for ASD has noted that although individuals with ASD can be resistant to touch, they are receptive to massage.[4,5] There are several factors that might help explain why massage is well received. Massage is intentional, systematic application of touch. This is something that a person can understand—especially when the sequence of techniques becomes predictable over time. This is often the case when massaging an infant. When infants first receive massage they often cry, yet the part of their body being massaged is relaxed.

With frequent exposure to massage, smiling replaces crying. Infants are unable to speak and make their needs known or communicate their perception that something feels unfamiliar. When they cry, yet the muscles of their arm or leg are relaxed, they are trying to communicate this confusion. The massage does not hurt, it feels good, but it is something new that the infant does not understand.

Like infants, individuals with ASD may not be able to express confusion about the various stimuli to which they are exposed. When they are able to regulate exposure to a stimulus, they create a coping mechanism. This coping can help them to ignore a stimulus they perceive as unpleasant, increase exposure to a pleasant stimulus, or filter the stimulus so that they have time to learn and understand it. Sensory therapies train an individual with ASD to learn, assess, and respond appropriately to stimuli. Most of the activities in sensory therapies train the sense of touch in an indirect manner. Massage and the systematic application of touch can help to directly train the sense of touch. Learning about the sense of touch can help to understand how this is possible.

3
Senses and the Nervous System

In order to understand how touch works, it is important to have a basic understanding of the way the nerves and muscles are structured and how they function. This chapter reviews how the sense of touch works, and how the body executes movement. This will help make clear how massage can have general benefits and also affect sensory processing issues associated with ASD. Movement of the body (motor skill) is accomplished by the interaction between muscles, skin, and nerves. These are the same body systems that are important in receiving and responding to massage and touch. That may help with understanding why individuals with ASD often have difficulty with motor skill.

NERVES AND ACTIONS

The nervous system is the information center of the body. It is a two-way communication system that regulates body functions: one aspect of the nervous system gathers information, the other makes things happen. This is made possible by *processing* or *integration*—how the nervous system understands information and responds in an appropriate way. A person who has sensory processing disorder may have a problem receiving, understanding, or responding to some type of stimulation. What is essentially a breakdown in communication of information can occur in many different places along this communication highway.

The *sensory* or *afferent* aspect of the nervous system gathers information in the form of stimulation from the surrounding environment and from internal organs. The signal from the stimulus is integrated and understood by messengers within the nervous system (*interneurons*). Based on the sensory information, the *motor* or *efferent* aspect of the nervous system sends a signal (*impulse*) to muscles or organs in the body on how to respond. This signal contains instructions to do something (*excitatory impulse*) or not do something (*inhibitory impulse*). This enables an organism to sense and act based on interaction with its surroundings. Non-sentient or simple organisms instinctively seek stimuli and react by instinct because they are not capable of conscious thought. Sentient or conscious organisms, like people or animals, also seek stimuli and react. But, they are different from non-sentient organisms because they are capable of reacting based on conscious decisions or instinct.

The nervous system has two parts: central and peripheral. The brain and spinal cord are considered the *central nervous system* (CNS). All nerves that are located outside the brain or spinal cord are considered the *peripheral nervous system* (PNS). In very basic terms, the CNS is responsible for receiving information, understanding it, and making decisions on how—or if—to act. Because this ability is vital to survival, the brain and spinal cord are protected internally by layers of tissue and externally by bone (skull and spinal column), fat tissues, fluids, and the skin.

The brain has several different regions that are specialized to regulate different functions of the body. Breathing, speech, purposeful movement and coordination are controlled by specific areas of the brain. Other areas are involved in attention, memory, understanding emotions, discerning meaning, and activities like organizing and sequencing. The ability to learn and pay attention involves specific brain centers that coordinate with other areas of the brain depending on what is being learned or requires attention. For example, children learning how to write their name would integrate verbal, visual, and motor skills with memories and sequencing. Different regions of the brain are also capable of *selective attention*. That is the ability of a person to focus on specific stimuli and ignore others that are present. The parts of the brain involved in memories depend on the content of the memory. For example, remembering the feeling of hitting a tennis ball with a racquet integrates motor skill, coordination, visual, and sensory areas of the brain.

The brain has an area dedicated to understanding sensations (*sensory cortex*) and also houses areas specifically for four of the five special senses (sight, hearing, smell, and taste). A web-like system of blood vessels weaves through and around brain tissues delivering oxygen and other nutrients and removing wastes. The CNS is also nourished and protected by cerebrospinal fluid. This fluid circulates between the layers of tissues in the brain and spinal cord to form a protective cushion. It is a clear liquid that contains protein and glucose to nourish the brain.

The tissues of the nervous system are made up of functioning and supporting cells. Functioning nerves that receive or send impulses are called *neurons*. There are neurons all over the body. All neurons have three parts: a part that receives impulses (*dendrite*), a central part known as the cell body (*soma*), and a part that sends impulses (*axon*). The positions and structure of these three parts of a neuron are different depending on the neuron's location in the body and specific functions. Supporting cells that nourish or protect the nerves come in different shapes and sizes. These cells are smaller than neurons, but outnumber actual neurons due to the needs of nervous system tissues.

The spinal cord is a large bundle of sensory and motor neurons that runs from the base of the brain (brainstem) to the lower back. It branches out at different heights to connect with the peripheral nerves. Like the brain, the spinal cord is bathed and protected by cerebrospinal fluid. The role of the spinal cord is to transmit nerve impulses or signals between the PNS and the brain.

The PNS is an enormous network of nerves. It is made up of sensory and motor nerves that reach from the spinal cord to tissues all over the inside and outside of the body. The sensory nerves receive information from the environment; the motor nerves stimulate muscles and glands in the body. A typical person does not consciously sense everything in the environment. Because there is a large amount of potential sensory input from the surroundings at any given time, all of it is not transmitted to the brain; therefore it is not consciously understood. This is a rather complex phenomenon called *action potential*. Basically this means that any type of stimulus must be strong enough to trigger a sensory or motor nerve impulse. When a sensory nerve impulse reaches the CNS, is processed, and triggers the response of motor neurons, it causes *physiological arousal*. The state of arousal is preparation for the body to act in some way depending on the sensory information. For example, a person may see a hot fudge sundae and start salivating in anticipation of taking a bite.

The motor nerves of the PNS can be divided into two systems: voluntary and involuntary. The *somatic* branch of the PNS controls voluntary movements like walking, reaching, turning, and bending. The internal organs of the body are controlled by the *autonomic* branch of the PNS. Organ functions like breathing, digestion, bowel movements, urination, and the beating of the heart are involuntary. They do not require conscious thought, but they are necessary for survival. Involuntary functions of the body change in response to a person's environment. There are two divisions of the autonomic branch of the PNS that increase or decrease physiological arousal.

Most anatomy students learn to differentiate the branches of the autonomic nervous system by identifying the *sympathetic* branch as *fight or flight* and the *parasympathetic* branch as *rest and digest*. The responses produced by the sympathetic and parasympathetic nervous system are instinctual. Basically these systems help the body to respond to stimuli and to preserve its resources by relaxation and nutrition. Based on sensory input, the nervous system sends impulses to organs of the endocrine system and to muscles. The endocrine system releases certain types of hormones depending on the stimulus. The skeletal muscles (which produce movement), as well as the heart (cardiac) muscle and the smooth muscles that control internal organs also contract or relax in reaction to the stimulus.

The sympathetic branch of the autonomic nervous system involves a series of excitatory and inhibitory responses that increase physiological arousal in response to stress or perceived danger. The eyes dilate, breathing and heart rate get faster, the muscles of the arms and legs tighten, and body hair literally stands up. Digestion slows down and the body tries to conserve fluids. A sudden or short-term stressor enhances the ability to think of the big picture, but interferes with the ability to focus on small details. Through sympathetic nervous system arousal the body is in essence trying to do three things:

- increase the ability to understand what is going on by dilating the eyes, stimulating hair, and shifting the brain's ability to focus

- prepare the body to run away by stimulating breathing, heart rate, and muscles

- stop any unnecessary body functions by stopping digestion and conserving fluids.

This helps to explain why a person who is suddenly scared may urinate or defecate spontaneously. The body is trying to get rid of excess waste that could interfere with the ability to run away.

The fight or flight response can kick in if a person is confronted with real or imagined danger, or psychosocial stress. A person might have similar physiological arousal if they saw a bear in their yard, watched a scary movie, or were about to propose marriage. Despite the prevalence of psychological, social, and physical stress in human life, the exact mechanisms that cause a person to respond to stress are not well understood. What is clear is that somehow physical and psychological functions deteriorate with prolonged exposure to stress. Prolonged physical or psychological stress can cause damage to the body because of the toll it takes on the organs of the body. If the body does not have adequate resources or the ability to respond to danger, it can shut down in some way.[6] Thankfully, the body can be trained to respond to stress or danger in a healthy way. Regular exercise helps to improve the function of the muscles and internal organs by conditioning them to small amounts of controlled stress.

Education—and if necessary psychological counseling—can help a person learn to cope with stressors. In many ways, any sensory therapy is an educational opportunity to help an individual with ASD to recognize what is a stressor and what is not.

The parasympathetic branch of the autonomic nervous system has the opposite effect of the sympathetic branch. It prepares the body to rest by constricting the pupils to filter out light, slowing heart rate and breathing, decreasing blood pressure, and increasing salivation, mucus production, and digestion. The brain is able to focus on small details and comprehend complex problems. Parasympathetic nervous system arousal attempts to return the body to normal by helping it to heal in three ways:

- *relaxation*, by filtering out light, slowing heart rate and breathing

- *nutrition*, by increasing saliva and mucus to promote digestion

- *repair*, which occurs when the body has adequate rest and nutrition for tissues.

Although the parasympathetic process sounds somewhat passive, it is not. All aspects of relaxation involve an excitatory or inhibitory stimulus. To facilitate digestion, blood is directed away from muscles and towards the internal organs. This gives some credence to the assumption that a person should wait one hour after eating before they go swimming. If the body is busy digesting, it will not have enough blood to deliver oxygen to muscles needed to help them swim.

As a child grows, they encounter various external stimuli. Some require a response while others do not. A person with sensory problems must understand what a stimulus is, if it is potentially dangerous or important, and/or if it requires a response. Essentially this is *coping*, which is learned by interacting as well as trial and error. Coping can be instinctual or intentional based on experience, memory, emotions, or cognitive knowledge. When sensory or motor communication breaks down, it interferes with the ability to cope.

Any damage to sensory neurons, interneurons, motor neurons, or the tissues of the brain or spinal cord, or a problem with blood flow to the brain would interfere in some way with body function. That is because it breaks down the chain of communication of information between the body and the brain. The amount of damage and the specific nervous system structure affected will show a specific sign or symptom related to sensation, organ function, or movement. Impairment of sensory neurons (as well as the nerves responsible for transmitting impulses related to sight, hearing, taste, and smell) would deprive the central nervous system of information. Damage to motor neurons would affect the ability to move as well as the functions of internal organs. Finally, damage to the brain or interneurons would interfere with the integration of information between sensory and motor neurons.

A child's nervous system grows and is trained by exposure to stimuli through education and activity. It takes practice to develop gross and fine motor skills because it requires coordination between nerves and muscles. It takes time to learn what is "good" and "bad" in physical surroundings, behavior, and social relationships. Children learn when it is appropriate to act using instinct or reason by learning to identify appropriate behavior and understanding information received through the senses.

SENSES

The body has several different sensory systems. They give information to the brain about what is going on inside the body and outside the body in the surrounding environment. Basic sensations involve information that can be transmitted to the brain from different systems in the body. The information is gathered from sensory receptors. It is converted to electrical impulse (*stimulus*) that is sent to the brain by sensory nerves or neurons. The body has a general sense that it can get from two types of sensory neurons: visceral and somatic.

- A *visceral sensory neuron* gathers information from within the body through sensations from the internal organs. It relays information to the brain about body functions like hunger, thirst, or the need to urinate. Awareness of these sensations occurs in the first few years of life.

- A *somatic sensory neuron* gathers information from the skin, muscles, and joints. It tells the brain about body position, movement, or temperature. Somatic sensory neurons are also involved in the sense of touch.

- *Touch* is one of the body's special senses, along with sight, hearing, smell, and taste. These senses work together to give the central nervous system (the brain and spinal cord) information about the self and the environment. The special senses play a vital role in helping to keep the body safe and healthy. They are also important communication.

The special senses

The sense of *sight* collects information about the environment. The eyes see the surroundings. They collect information about the space, position, and relationships between the objects and people. Motion and speed are concepts that a person understands through seeing. Sight also gives proprioceptive information about the position of the body. The sense of sight involves light that is converted into nerve impulses which are transmitted to the visual cortex in the brain. The understanding or comprehension of what a person sees occurs in the brain. Sight is important for navigation, safety, and communication. It helps a person to make decisions about where to move, walk, or reach. Reading visual cues also helps a person form interpersonal relationships. Sight also helps keep a person out of danger and protect others. Sometimes a visual stimulus causes a reflex or unconscious reaction. Throwing an object towards a person's face will cause them to move out of the way without thinking. Seeing an animal in the middle of the road might cause a driver of a car to press the brake pedal. In both cases, the person reacts to a change in their surroundings because of information that was relayed to their brain through open eyes.

The anatomical structure of the eye enables the brain and body to regulate sensory information. The pupil of the eye constricts to filter out light or dilates to bring in more light. The eyelids can also be partially or fully closed. Squinting is one way to limit sensory input from sight. Often squinting happens spontaneously when a person is suddenly exposed to bright lights. Over time the eyes adapt to the light and the lids relax to the open position. Partially closing one or both eyes, or squinting, is common in individuals with ASD.

The sense of *hearing* collects sound stimulus from the environment and the self. Sounds have different pitch, quality, tone, and volume. These different qualities help to identify what a sound is, the location and the source of a sound. Over time a person also learns what a sound means. The sense of hearing involves conversion of sound waves to nerve impulses. Hearing involves three parts of the ear: outer, middle, and inner. Sound waves flow through the outer ear to the tympanic membrane or ear drum in the middle ear. This membrane vibrates in response to the sound waves. It also causes three little bones (hammer, anvil, and stirrup) to vibrate, sending the vibration further into the ear to the chambers of the inner ear. These vibrations are converted to nerve impulses which are transmitted to the auditory cortex in the brain.

The ears serve two purposes: hearing and proprioception. There are two structures in the inner ear that are important for proprioception: semilunar canals and Eustachian tubes. The inner ear contains a labyrinth of tubes and compartments that are filled with fluid and lined with tiny hairs. The *semilunar canals* are a portion of this structure that collect information about vertical and horizontal movement of the head. The *Eustachian tubes* travel from the ear to the back of the throat. They can be opened to regulate air pressure within the ear. They also drain excess mucus from the ear. When the Eustachian tubes are obstructed, it can affect hearing and balance.

Hearing plays an important role in communication, relationships, education, and entertainment. Interpersonal communication involves talking and listening. Hearing helps children to form words when they are learning to talk. Children listen to others speak and then imitate by speaking while they listen to the sound of their own voice. Hearing is important in relationships. Talking and listening is how we learn what other people think or feel. Understanding the qualities of a person's voice also helps us to understand what a person is trying to say. Sometimes the same words can have different meanings depending on a person's tone of voice. A person might yell "Oh my gosh!" if they are happily surprised or if something frightening just happened. Listening to music or the sounds on videos, film, or television are forms of education and entertainment. The use of bells, sirens, and whistles in communities is evidence that hearing is important for personal safety.

Unlike the eyes, the body is not able to independently close the ears to limit sensory input from sounds. The hands can be pressed over the ears or the tragus can be pressed over the opening of the ear canal to limit sound. Devices can be used to shut out sounds, including ear plugs placed in the ear or noise-reduction headphones worn over the ear. Humming, singing, or talking can be used to overwhelm sounds from the surroundings or other people. Loud or unpleasant sounds are not easy to ignore. Individuals with ASD are often sensitive to sound, including background noises or pleasant noises. This may happen because of difficulty discerning between different sounds and filtering out background noises. The hum of an electrical appliance might appear overwhelmingly loud compared to a person standing next to it who is speaking.

When someone is unable to discern different sounds, it can be frustrating and difficult to focus attention on important sounds as well as other sensory stimuli. That is why it is harder to have a conversation near the checkout counter of a busy grocery store than in the car on the way home. Announcements over the loud speaker, people talking close by, beeping of the scanner, rustling or clanking of items as they are placed on the conveyor, and even the motor of the conveyor can be overwhelming when an individual with ASD tries to take it all in. A typical person learns to focus on specific important sounds and ignore all of the others. Learning to pay attention to specific sounds and ignore others is how a person is able to regulate the sense of hearing.

The senses of smell and taste are closely linked. The sense of *smell* starts with airflow through the nose. The nasal cavity has sensory receptors that respond to chemicals in the air. There are millions of olfactory sensors that project into the nasal cavity. The airborne chemicals bind to these neurons which creates a nerve impulse. This impulse travels to the olfactory cortex in the brain as well as areas of the brain that are involved with emotions and memories. That is why certain smells seem to have connections with emotions or past events.

Smelling vanilla is usually associated with pleasant feelings. Coincidentally, it can make people think of chocolate chip cookies (which use vanilla as an ingredient). A person may not consciously make the connection between vanilla to chocolate chip cookie to sitting in the kitchen and having a snack that mother or grandmother baked. The smell just sparks a warm, cared-for feeling. The sense of smell is a primal sense that can have important affects on the subconscious. The sense of smell is usually weak when someone has a cold or allergies because mucus builds up in the nose and blocks the nasal passages. Smell can also be affected by certain medications, ear infections, or an injury. Because the senses of smell and taste are understood in the same areas of the brain, impairment of the sense of smell influences the ability to taste. Therefore, inability to smell can affect eating habits, food choices, and even general interest in food.

Sensory information about *taste* comes from the taste buds that line the tongue, cheeks, and roof of the mouth. It also comes from smell. There are several thousand taste buds that are skin cells which are specialized to be able to discern different tastes. Taste involves flavor, acidity, and texture. Flavors are usually perceived as complex, but there are four basic flavors: sweet, bitter, salty, and sour. (It is possible that a fifth flavor exists—umami—which comes from savory foods and proteins.) Taste also involves a basic chemical sense that helps to distinguish flavors that are spicy or acidic. The mouth also has temperature sensors (*thermoreceptors*) which give the ability to distinguish between a food that is chemically hot, such as a jalapeno pepper, and a food that has a hot temperature, such as a baked potato.

Taste is understood through a combination of the taste buds, sensory nerves on the lips (*mechanoreceptors*), as well as the actions of chewing with the muscles of the mouth and jaw. Stimulation of taste buds involves chemicals from food that are dissolved in saliva. Taste buds open to receive these chemicals and this triggers a nerve impulse. The nerve impulse is sent to the brain where it combines with the smell (olfactory) sensors. That is how smell and taste are interlinked.

In addition to flavors, foods have texture. The texture of foods ranges from liquid to solid, with many distinctions in between. Liquid or gel-like foods can be easily swallowed. The texture does not change much when food combines with saliva in the mouth. Foods that are fibrous, gummy, crunchy, or dense undergo changes in texture during mastication (chewing and swallowing). While the texture of pudding or pureed food does not change between the time it passes the lips and is swallowed, the texture of a carrot, jelly bean, pretzel, or piece of cheddar cheese will change substantially during mastication. A typical child learns to understand mastication and changes in food texture as it progresses from baby food to solid foods. A child who has difficulty with sensory processing may not learn this concept as easily. Spitting out food after chewing may be due to sensitivity to changes in food texture during mastication. Similarly sometimes the flavor or acidity of food can overwhelm the ability to sense a food's texture. Chocolate pudding is very flavorful compared to plain yogurt but the texture is nearly identical. The flavor and the sugar in chocolate pudding make it seem tastier than plain yogurt, which decreases attention to the texture. Eating foods that are not necessarily flavorful but have a distinct texture can also be unpleasant.

The way the brain understands the texture of food is similar to the way it understands the sense of touch. The complexity that is required to taste food may help to shed light on the difficulties many individuals with ASD have with feeding. When a person cannot smell or taste food, the sense of the texture of food becomes very obvious. Foods may be limited or ignored because of the flavor or acidity but it may also be due to the perception of the texture as unpleasant or uninteresting. There is a distinct relationship between the texture of food and the sense of touch because of the way touch is perceived.

The senses of smell and taste can be regulated by removing exposure to the stimulus. When people do not like a smell, they instinctively press their nostrils closed. A person who does not like the taste of food can take it out of the mouth. The ability to filter, regulate, or remove sensory input through the eyes, ears, nose, or mouth is a benefit and a potential problem. It is a benefit because it can easily remove exposure to an unpleasant stimulus. It is a potential problem because the senses are trained through exposure to stimuli. Training the body's sense of touch and general senses is more problematic because it is very difficult to filter out this type of sensory information.

The sense of touch

Touch is contact with something or someone. It is a sense that carries meaning. Touch is also called the tactile sense. The things that individuals choose to touch, how they respond to touch, the way they touch others and how they like to be touched are very personal. Touch is subjective to each and every person. Simply shaking hands with several different people gives a good idea of how differently people touch each other and are receptive to touch.

The sense of touch serves two basic functions: discrimination and protection. *Discrimination* is the ability to tell the difference between things. Through touch a person can understand what an object is based on shape, size, texture, weight, position, and temperature. With touch a person can distinguish how that object is different from other things. For example, a zucchini and a flashlight are approximately the same size and shape. However, they can be distinguished based on texture, surface features, weight, and temperature. When two objects share one tactile characteristic, other tactile characteristics help a person differentiate between the two. Table 3.1 gives examples of objects that are different but share one tactile characteristic. Each column of the table shows different objects that share similar tactile characteristics. Touch and discernment help a person to learn the difference.

Table 3.1 Tactile characteristics

Reference object	Pencil	Softball	Plastic bucket	Textbook	Ice cube
Tactile characteristic					
Shape	String bean	Tennis ball	Basket	Picture frame	Ring box
Size	Hair clip	Grapefruit	Basketball	Binder	Golf ball
Texture	Stick	Leather jacket	CD case	Memo board	Glass
Weight	Lipstick	Gym shoe	Pitcher	Potted plant	Shot glass
Temperature	Wood block	Leather belt	Mop handle	Ceramic plate	Snowball

A zucchini and a flashlight also serve different functions: one is edible, the other is a tool. Like the sensory information from the other special senses, children learn through touch how different things feel which helps identify and discern objects. They learn that a circle has smooth edges and a triangle or rectangle has sharp corners. They integrate this knowledge with visual and auditory information to understand what different objects are and how they can be used. This helps them to learn not to try to eat a flashlight or light the room with a zucchini.

Touch also helps individuals to learn the boundaries of their own body by helping them discriminate the difference between the self and the surrounding environment. Touch can give a sense of space to a person in the same way that a cat uses its whiskers to figure out whether it can safely fit through the pet door. The cat's whiskers are as wide as its body so if the whiskers bend when it puts its head through the door, the cat instinctively knows that its body would not fit. A human's sense of space and boundaries comes from many different sensory receptors all over the body. Someone sitting on a chair is able to understand where his body ends and the bench begins because he can feel the chair. Pressure, position, and sensory receptors in the skin and muscles all work together to give the person this understanding. Children learn about the physical limits of their own body through touch and movement. Essentially they experiment in order to understand their environment. This helps them develop their sense of awareness of the body in space (*kinesthetic awareness*), understand the position of their body (*proprioception*), and learn about their environment.

Individuals with sensory problems may kick or hit out of aggression or frustration. It may also be an attempt to get sensory input to help understand who they are and what is around them. Biting is another behavior that may be related to tactile sensing. Most children try to taste objects—even inedible objects—in an experiential way. Biting or squeezing things helps to understand texture and density of an object.

Biting or chewing inedible objects may be a way to evaluate or experiment in order to understand the density or texture of an object in an unusual way.

Like the other special senses, touch plays a role in *protection* by helping the body to avoid harm. Sensory information can alert the body to danger from extreme heat, cold, or even caustic substances. When a person comes in contact with something that is potentially damaging, he or she can withdraw. This helps protect the body from harm. The sense of touch is thought to be the first of the special senses to develop in utero.

Touch is unique among the special senses because of the way that information about touch is relayed to the brain. Sight, hearing, taste, and smell all involve sensory information that comes into the head. Touch is more complicated because it is perceived all over the body. Thousands of sensors can give information to the brain at any moment in time. The sense of touch simultaneously evaluates multiple characteristics of the object including shape, size, texture, weight and temperature. This evaluation also includes an assessment of whether the object being touched is potentially dangerous or harmful. With time and practice the brain learns to understand what the sensations are, what they mean, and what response (if any) is required.

Although there are touch sensors all over the surface of the skin, they are very organized. Sensory nerves travel to the spinal cord in a hierarchical and logical fashion. Sensory (afferent) nerves from the arms and shoulders enter the upper part of the spinal cord. Trunk nerves enter the middle of the spinal cord and nerves from the legs enter the lower part of the spinal cord. From the spinal cord some—but not all— nerve impulses may travel up to the brain.

At any given time, the human body is touching multiple things. A person who is sitting in a chair reading a book would be touching the book, chair, clothing, and shoes. These sensations are felt from different places in the body and sent to the brain to help the body understand position. The brain makes conscious and unconscious decisions in response to the sense of touch. When touching an object is uncomfortable or unpleasant, the body tends to withdraw. A person may relax or move toward a comfortable or pleasant touch. The pressure, temperature, and qualities of touch can vary considerably in terms of how it is perceived.

Certain types of touch can overpower other sensations. When that happens the brain learns to pay attention to important stimuli. People lying on the beach might be aware of the sun's heat on their body. If an insect lands on their leg they will become acutely aware of the light touch of the insect. This awareness will replace the feeling of warmth from the sun. A typical person is able to adapt to different touch stimuli and ignore any sensation that is not potentially threatening or requiring an action. Someone with a sensory disorder may not be able to differentiate between the various sensations. The collective message to the brain is confusing. Learning how the brain understands touch will help explain how this can occur.

4 Sensations and Awareness

There are two basic ways that touch is understood by the brain: *tactile sensation* and *kinesthetic awareness*. Different sensory organs in the nervous system are specialized to feel specific types of touch. The concept of kinesthetic awareness includes input from many different types of sensors that are located all over the body. Kinesthetic awareness is discussed later in the chapter.

TACTILE SENSATION

Tactile sensation is a term that refers to the perception of touch that is made possible by different types of sensors located in the skin, muscles, and tendons. These sensors are specialized to receive specific types of information. There are three basic types of sensations: temperature, pressure, and pain. Each sensation is perceived with a special sensor: temperature—*thermoreceptors*, pressure—*mechanoreceptors*, and pain—*nociceptors*. The combination of sensory input from more than one type of sensor helps to make the typical person capable of discerning many different types of touch.

Brushing therapy and joint compression are used in sensory therapy to improve tactile sensations and kinesthetic awareness. For brushing to be effective, a stiff-bristled brush is needed to provide a deep sensation. This can be irritating to sensitive skin. A medium- or soft-bristled brush may be less irritating, but pressing hard with the supple bristles just bends the bristles rather than increasing the pressure put on the sensory receptors in the skin. Stroking techniques of massage offer a possible alternative. The sensory therapy joint compression technique involves pressing the bones of a joint closer together. This naturally occurs in the knees and ankles during walking. It is theorized that this stimulates the sensory receptors in the joints. Massage also stimulates the same sensory receptors because massage is applied to muscles and connective tissues that cross the joints. An added benefit of massage is that there are additional sensory receptors in the muscles and skin that can be stimulated by kneading, compression, percussion, gliding strokes, and stretching techniques used in massage.

Thermoreceptors and temperature

The body has a general sense of temperature from the air and environment. An area of the brain called the hypothalamus regulates internal body temperature. If a person gets too warm, it stimulates the body to sweat to help cool internal temperature. If a person gets too cold, the body shivers.

Shivering is unconscious muscle contractions that help to provide heat within the body.

Thermoreceptors in the various layers of the skin sense changes in temperature. They are found on the skin all over the body and in the mouth and are specialized to sense either warm or cold. Warm sensors are located closer to the surface of the skin; cold sensors are deeper. Different areas of the skin are more sensitive to temperature because of the number of thermoreceptors contained in that area. Thermoreceptors respond to a change in temperature. Shifting of temperature from warm to cold or cold to warm sends a signal to the brain. Picking up an ice cube causes an immediate sense that the ice cube is cold. That is because it is colder than room temperature and body temperature. Picking up a deck of cards would not activate thermoreceptors because the cards are closer to room temperature. People can safely tolerate exposure to different temperatures. But severe temperatures or prolonged exposure of the skin to moderately severe temperatures can cause injury.

Mechanoreceptors and pressure

Mechanoreceptors sense pressure. That includes pressure that is applied to the body as well as pressure applied to objects and surfaces. There are different types of mechanoreceptors that sense a change in force applied to tissues of the body. They are specialized to sense different types of pressure including: movement, vibration, deep touch, light touch, and sustained pressure. Different mechanoreceptors are also specialized to adapt over time. They can either adapt quickly or slowly. Fastadapting mechanoreceptors begin to respond to the stimulus immediately but then quickly cease. This plays an important role in the adaptation to touch. Slow-adapting mechanoreceptors also respond immediately to a stimulus but they continue to respond until the stimulus is removed.

Mechanoreceptors are located in different areas of the skin and muscles. Some are close to the surface of the skin, while others lie deep within muscles or joints. Mechanoreceptors close to the surface of the skin (*cutaneous*) are specialized to sense light touch and movement, while those that are located deeper within the skin or in the muscles sense heavier pressure and joint position. The roles of some of the different mechanoreceptors overlap in what they are capable of sensing and how they adapt to stimuli.

- *Hair follicle receptors* are sensory receptors which are located on the skin next to hair follicles. In addition to the hair on the head, pubic, and underarm, the body has fine hair on the face, arms, legs, and torso. Hair follicle receptors are fast-adapting mechanoreceptors that give information about movement. This can include movement of the body or movement of something around the body, like a brush or a breeze from a fan. Movement causes the fine hairs to sway which stimulates the hair follicle receptors. This is similar to the cat using its whiskers to fit through a door, but on a larger level. The swaying of the hairs away from the direction of movement gives the body a sense of direction. Hair follicles are attached to the skin with a tiny muscle (arrector pili). When this muscle contracts, the hair becomes erect. This is caused by stimulation by the sympathetic nervous system in the fight or flight response or when a person is cold.

- *Meissner's corpuscles* are located close to the surface of the skin. They are located all over the skin but are important on hairless areas like the fingertips, lips, and nipples. They are fast adapting and sense light touch and slow vibration. Meissner's corpuscles help give the fingertips, lips, and nipples extreme sensitivity.

- *Ruffini endings* are found in the subcutaneous layer of the skin and the tissue that surrounds the joints (*joint capsule*). Also called *Ruffini's end organs*, these mechanoreceptors are slow adapting. They sense vibration, stretching of the skin, and may also sense deep pressure and heat. Because of their location and ability to sense pressure and stretching, they contribute to proprioceptive awareness.

- *Pacinian corpuscles* are located in the skin and some mucus membranes. They are located in the subcutaneous layer of the skin and other connective tissues. They are very sensitive, fast-adapting mechanoreceptors that can sense position because they are stimulated by vibration, pressure, and tension. Pacinian corpuscles located in tissues of the joints also play a role in proprioception.

- *Merkel's discs* are located in clusters all over the skin including on mucus membranes, on hairy skin, and the glabrous skin of the hands and feet, and on the fingertips. They are slow-adapting mechanoreceptors that sense form and texture because they are sensitive to pressure, intensity of pressure, and vibration. Merkel's discs likely contribute to kinesthetic awareness. They may help the body to learn and remember movement. Since they are sensitive and slow adapting, that may explain why many individuals with ASD seek deep pressure. Merkel's discs would be activated by weighted vests or pressure garments.

The smooth, hair-free skin on the palms of the hands and soles of the feet (*glabrous*) does not contain hair follicles. Therefore, it does not have hair follicle receptors. But hands and feet do have a large number of different types of sensory receptors. These areas of the body are particularly sensitive because they contain large numbers of *free nerve endings*. These sensory receptors are nonspecific and may be fast or slow adapting. They serve multiple purposes because they do not respond to a specific type of stimulus. Rather, they work as multipurpose mechanoreceptors as well as thermoreceptors and nociceptors. Since they are not specialized they are able to gather information about many different qualities of an object simultaneously. They coordinate their sensations with other types of sensory receptors to evaluate various qualities of touch.

Muscles and tendons contain sensory structures that give the body information about the length of muscles or the load on muscles. In plain language that means the sensors assess and respond to muscles that are overstretched or overweighted. Length or stretching of muscles is sensed by intrafusal muscle fibers called *muscle spindles*. These structures run alongside contractile muscle fibers but they do not contract. Rather they are sensors that gather information about the length of muscles. Muscle spindles deter muscles from overstretching by stimulating an overstretched muscle to contract. This helps to explain why a person trying to touch their toes may feel a twinge in the back of their leg. If the hamstring muscles are tight, reaching too far will be perceived as dangerous by the muscle spindles. The twinge feeling occurs when the overstretched hamstring muscle fibers are stimulated to contract by the muscle spindles.

Muscle spindles also sense how fast a muscle is stretched. Gentle and slow stretching of muscles does not activate muscle spindles. Gentle stretching helps to relax tight and sore muscles. It is not likely to cause damage, so the body senses it is an appropriate activity. Bouncing while stretching—as in ballistic stretching—can increase flexibility but it can also be dangerous. That is because the muscle spindles receive two danger messages: too far, too fast. This may stimulate more muscle fibers to contract simultaneously which can strain the muscle.

The activity of muscle spindles is not conscious. The time between the stimulus and reaction is very short because the nerve impulse does not travel to the brain. Rather it travels from the muscle spindle to the spinal cord and back to the muscle fibers. A quick reaction is necessary to help the body stay safe. Because muscle spindles are very sensitive they are important in reflexes. This is demonstrated by the quadriceps (patellar) tendon test that is usually performed as part of a medical exam. Hitting the tendon (below the kneecap) with a mallet causes overstretching in the quadriceps muscles. The muscle spindle causes contraction of the quadriceps muscle which is why the knee extends or straightens.

Another sensory structure located in muscles and tendons is the *Golgi tendon organ*. These are small structures found in tendons and near where muscle fibers and tendons converge. Golgi tendon organs sense too much weight or overload on working muscles. It senses the load as dangerous and stimulates the working muscle(s) to relax. A person trying to lift a heavy box might drop it suddenly. If the box is too heavy, the Golgi tendon organ sends a message that the arm muscles are overloaded. This stimulates the muscles to relax, which causes them to lower or drop the box. This may involve conscious thought—or not—depending on the difference between the strength of the muscle and the weight or load. In other words, a person can successfully lift something that is slightly heavy but not something that is extremely heavy in relation to their muscle strength. They would either fail to lift the extremely heavy object at all or drop it during the lifting phase. Training can help muscles adapt to overloading, but it must be progressive in order to avoid stimulating the Golgi tendon organs.

Different categories of mechanoreceptors are capable of receiving different types of pressure information: deep, light, movement, vibration, sustained pressure as well as the length of and load on muscles. The sensory stimuli received by the Ruffini endings, Pacinian corpuscles, muscle spindles and Golgi tendon organs contribute to the awareness of body position.[7] The sensory stimuli received by hair follicle receptors, Meissner's corpuscles, Merkel's discs, and free nerve endings help, through touch, to identify aspects about the environment. Collectively all mechanoreceptors contribute to an overall sense of the self and the environment.

It is possible that differences noted in the touch-sensitivities across the ASD spectrum may be caused by alterations in patterns of arousal or sensitivity of one or more of these types of mechanoreceptors. It is also possible that the extreme volume of sensory information that is perceived through the sense of touch and pressure causes sensory dysfunction. When the sense of touch is impaired—whatever the explanation—the result is either increased or decreased sensitivity.

Fast-adapting mechanoreceptors require continual stimulation to sense pressure; they would be stimulated by repeated touch like tapping or stroking. This type of stimulus would not be felt by slow-adapting mechanoreceptors. Likewise, the stimulus of slow-adapting mechanoreceptors by holding or squeezing would not be felt by fast-adapting mechanoreceptors. These specific sensors for different types of touch may help to explain why some individuals with ASD are categorized as hyper- or hypo-sensitive to touch.

Hyper-sensitive individuals may have over-reactive fast-adapting mechanoreceptors. Basically that means their threshold for feeling a repeated stimulus is quite low. The perception of a single tap on the shoulder may feel like repeated taps or even a punch. They may have increased awareness of the sensation of fabric as clothing moves across their skin when they move. They may seek stillness because any movement may provide substantial sensory input from hair follicles and other mechanoreceptors that is overwhelming. In these situations, slow, sustained touch may be best tolerated because the increased touch sensitivity is closely related to the perception of pain.

Conversely, a person who is hypo-sensitive may have under-reactive fast-adapting mechanoreceptors. They would have a higher threshold need to feel a stimulus. They might not respond to a light tap on the shoulder, but instead require several taps, or a tap with deeper pressure. They may respond well to wearing a weighted or pressure vest which would provide continuous stimulus of their slow-adapting mechanoreceptors. This individual may move about a lot by jumping or spinning in order to provide adequate sensory input to their fast-adapting mechanoreceptors. For this individual, vigorous or deep touch would likely be tolerated best because it goes over the sensory threshold.

For an individual with sensitivities to touch, learning to pay attention to an important stimulus and ignore other stimuli is problematic. Training their nervous system to sense and perceive touch is a logical first step. This helps them to understand the difference between stimulation, sensation, and pain.

Nociceptors and pain

The sense of pain is a general response to stimuli which alerts the body to potential harm. Despite the many different types of pain that are known to exist in humans, pain is not well understood. Pain can be caused by an unpleasant sensation or actual damage to the tissues of the body. It involves sensory input from nociceptors. *Nociceptors* are free nerve endings in the skin and subcutaneous tissue. They include both fast- and slow-adapting sensors. It is unclear whether nociceptors work in coordination with other sensory receptors, or are capable of independently sensing temperature or pressure qualities that may be harmful. What is known is that there are somatic (body) and visceral (internal organ) nociceptors that send impulses to the central nervous system in response to real or potential harm.

Scientific research has not been able to clearly identify the pathway by which pain signals are received and comprehended by the brain. It is thought to be a gate system: an unpleasant stimulus is sent to the brain which closes off (inhibits) attention to any other stimulus.[8] A person who stubs his toe and then bangs his elbow as he reaches down to grab his foot would find that the pain was worse in either the toe or the elbow, but not equally bad in both. This also helps explain why an icepack or a heat compress can relieve a muscle ache. Pain might also be a complicated interaction between the endocrine, nervous, and immune systems.[9] Pain displaying behaviors, such as crying, yelling, or writhing, are learned behaviors that have strong roots in cultures. Pain is a subjective, but very real phenomenon.

Temperature, injury, chemical changes in the body, and even tension of tissues can cause pain. A topical burn on the skin can be painful; so can cutting the skin with a sharp object. Inflammation is a chemical change in the body that can cause pain. Stretching or squeezing the skin or muscle, moving a joint beyond its range of motion, or wearing a belt that is too tight can be painful. Pain plays an important role in alerting the brain to something that could cause the body harm. But it also can result from a non-threatening stimulus. Experiencing pain helps a person learn about potential dangers. It can also impact preference for touch. Tickling someone with a feather may be pleasant for one person yet painful for another. It is not dangerous or threatening, but the sense is unpleasant so the act of tickling stimulates the nociceptors to send a signal to the brain. The ability to cope with different intensities of pain is called *pain tolerance*. It is not known whether a person has a different perception of the pain or has a higher stimulus threshold before the nociceptors send a message to the brain, but the identification of people who cannot feel pain or are indifferent to pain suggests that this may be a possible physiological explanation.

Pain has different qualities. It can be dull or sharp; local or widespread, short-term (acute) or long-term (chronic) in duration. Dull pain is usually described as an ache; sharp pain is often described as shooting or pointed. Sharp pain is perceived as more specific and intense than dull pain and is often more localized. Muscle soreness after a workout would be perceived as dull pain, but an intense sudden muscle cramp would feel like a sharp pain. Pain is local when it is felt in a specific area and widespread when it is perceived in multiple areas of the body. Burning a finger on a hot stove produces local pain, but sunburn from a day at the beach would cause widespread pain. The stimulus and the tissues affected by that stimulus influence the quality of pain. A bout of appendicitis or a sprained ankle can cause acute pain. Low back pain is described as chronic pain when it is felt over several months and has no known physical or physiological cause.

An unusual attribute of pain is referral. When pain is felt at a site that is far from the stimulus, it is called *referred pain*. A person with gallstones may feel pain near their right shoulder blade. Pressing an injured area of muscle may cause pain in an area several inches away (see Chapter 7, "Neuromuscular massage," for a discussion of myofascial trigger points). Regardless of the source of pain or quality of pain, it is unpleasant and can interfere with a person's ability to function.

KINESTHETIC AWARENESS

Kinesthetic awareness is the understanding of the position of the body. Sometimes called *proprioception*, this information is perceived by several different sensory structures located throughout the body. Sensors in the inner ear (semilunar canals) provide feedback about the position of the head. Mechanoreceptors in the skin and muscles give an understanding of the position of the body by collecting information about stretching of skin, joint movement, and muscle tension. Together these sensory structures (called the *vestibular system*) work together to give the brain information about the relationship of the body to the surrounding environment. When the body is in motion, the brain gets information about the position, speed, and coordination of the head, arms, legs, and torso. When individuals receive information from any of their senses, they can respond or adapt to their surroundings.

Vision also contributes to kinesthetic awareness because it gives information about the environment and the head's orientation within that environment. Vision helps to understand direction and spatial relationships. It is easier to touch the nose with a finger when the eyes are open because you can see your nose and the direction your hand is moving. If individuals are unable to see their nose or hand, they lack an important aspect of kinesthetic awareness so they may miss and touch the mouth or the forehead. Impairment of one sense heightens awareness of other senses. When the eyes are closed, the senses of hearing and smell are more obvious. With practice, a person can identify direction and aspects of the surroundings by hearing or smelling when they cannot see. Sounds are different when a door is open versus when it is closed. Smells have a source, and it is possible to trace the source of a strong scent without looking. The popcorn stand at a movie theater or a barbecue at the park or beach is easy to find because the body can use information from the eyes, nose, and ears.

Kinesthetic awareness is influenced by the sensitivity of different joints to changes in position. The joints of the body that are closer to the trunk are less sensitive to position changes than the joints in the hands, ankles, and feet.[10] The differences in joint position sensitivity are logical and necessary. It is logical, because the body cannot pay attention to or understand too many stimuli, especially when the stimulus is not potentially dangerous. It is necessary because there is more potential for a change in position of the hands, ankles, or feet to cause harm (e.g. tripping, spraining an ankle) than a shift in position of the hip or shoulder. In other words, the ability to walk is affected by a person's balance. Misplacement of the entire leg would be caused by a deviation in the action of the hip joint. Under normal circumstances it would not likely be dangerous, but could cause a change in direction. Conversely, misplacement of the foot would be caused by deviation in the action of joints in the ankle or foot. If the side of the foot lands on the ground instead of the sole of the foot, it could cause a person to fall. When a child learns to walk, kinesthetic awareness happens through trial and error as well as repetition. Coordination develops over time as the body grows and moves. Exercise and movement are associated with improved kinesthetic awareness as well as improved ability to balance.

A person with a typical sense of kinesthetic awareness is able to subconsciously understand the position and movement of their body. This sense is made possible by the interaction between the various aspects of the body's general sensory system, the special senses, and the vestibular system. Given the involvement of multiple forms of sensory input, it is possible to overload the kinesthetic perception by exposing it to multiple stimuli simultaneously. For example, spinning, jumping, or swinging give sensory stimulation through vision, touch, and vestibular function at the same time. This often shifts attention away from external stimuli because the body cannot rely on the stimulus to get a sense of space or location. Often, this also creates confusing internal sensations. For a typical child or an adult, feeling dizzy, nauseous, or unsteady is not pleasurable. But that may not be true for an individual with ASD. It is possible that the internal sensations may be interesting or create a way to withdraw from the surroundings. It is also possible that the sensory overload increases kinesthetic awareness, even if it is not purposeful.

Proprioception

In basic terms, bones provide the framework of the body and muscles produce the movement. The body is capable of moving because muscles contract to pull bones toward each other and then relax to let the bones go back to their original position. There are 206 bones in the human body. Different bones come together to form many different joints like the hip, knee, ankle, shoulder, elbow, and wrist. The joints in the body allow movement of the body in different directions. It is a simple—and complex—operation that is made possible because of special properties of muscles as well as integration of certain aspects of many different systems of the body. Some parts of muscles are primarily involved in maintaining posture. These muscle fibers gently shorten (contract) over a prolonged period of time to hold the body upright in standing or sitting positions. Movement requires the use of more muscles and muscle fibers than maintaining posture.

The human body is made up of different types of tissue. The four basic types of tissue are skin, muscles, nerves, and connective tissue. Muscles are made up two types of tissue: muscle fibers and connective tissue. Muscle tissue has special characteristics. Muscle fibers are: excitable, contractile, extensible, and elastic. In order for a muscle to contract, the nervous system sends a message (*stimulus*) to the muscles. This message tells the muscle to do one of two things. Muscles are capable of receiving and responding (*excitable*) to that stimulus. The muscle may respond by shortening (*contracting*) or stretching (*extending*). Muscles are also *elastic* because after contracting or extending, they are able to return to their original position.

Muscles are made up of many muscle fibers that consist of contractile tissue. The actual fibers perform the contraction (shortening) of muscles. Muscle fibers are grouped together and surrounded by layers of connective tissue (fascia). Fascia has many layers that create bundles of muscle fibers. Each muscle has many groupings of muscle fibers and fascia. Individual muscle fibers are arranged in groups which are surrounded by fascia. Bundles of muscle fibers are grouped together and surrounded by fascia, and then groups of bundles are grouped together and surrounded by fascia. These groups of bundles are enclosed by fascia to create the whole muscle. Ultimately the layers of fascia that surround the bundles of muscle fibers come together to create a tendon that connects the muscle to the bones. In addition to surrounding muscle fibers, fascia also runs throughout the body. Fascia surrounds organs, separates the body into compartments, connects bones to each other, and connects muscles to bones.

Fascia stretches and relaxes alongside the muscle fibers but fascia does not contract by itself. Fascia can become chronically shortened when muscles are not regularly moved or stretched. Tight fascia can interfere with normal movement of the body. Massage and stretching techniques can relieve tight fascia by a variety of stretching techniques.

Muscles are arranged around the body to allow movement in different directions. These directions are dictated by the structure of the bones that form joints. For example, the knee and elbow are hinge joints that can move forward and backward like a door. Most joint movement is made possible by coordinated contraction of several muscles at one time (synergists). Each movement of a joint has an opposite movement that is performed by the contraction of another set of muscles (antagonists). In other words, a person can bend or straighten their knee because they have the ability to contract two different groups of muscles. The organization of the nervous system helps with the cycle of muscle contraction and relaxation. If a muscle contracts, the antagonist muscle for that movement is stimulated to relax. When a person has muscle tightness, the joint gets stiff. The balance of strength between the tight muscle and the opposite (antagonist) muscle becomes uneven. The opposite muscle lacks strength to restore posture and the tight muscle cannot return to a proper resting length.

Muscles can become tight for a variety of reasons. The work of muscles is contraction. The contraction of muscles shortens the muscle fiber and surrounding fascia bringing the bones closer together. This is how any movement—walking, running, typing, writing—is performed by the body. Postural habits, exercise, as well as occupational and recreational activities use groups of muscles in different ways. Physical activity and exercise promote muscle growth through conditioning but they can also contribute to muscle injury. The frequency and duration of the activity, intensity of muscle effort (the load or weight on the muscles), and the repetitive movements associated with the activity have potential to condition or damage muscles used. For example, tennis and baseball both involve similar movements of the shoulder joint. The force needed to throw a baseball from the outfield to home plate is substantial compared to the force needed to hit a tennis ball (much of the ball's energy is absorbed by the racquet). Either activity could result in sore or tight muscles.

The essential body systems that produce movement are the skeleton, the nervous system, and the muscular system. Secondary systems of the body that contribute to movement include the respiratory and cardiovascular systems (to give the muscles oxygen), digestive system (to give the muscles food to use as fuel), lymphatic and renal systems (to remove wastes), and the endocrine system (which helps carry messages between the various body systems in response to information it receives from the nervous system). Four of the special senses (sight, sound, touch, and hearing) are also involved in that they help the body move safely in relation to the environment. Basically, almost the entire body is involved in movement on some level.

Sensation is important in movement. A person must have kinesthetic awareness to be able to move the body in a purposeful manner and in a safe manner within their surrounding environment. They also must be aware of when they are moving and when they are still. This can be problematic in someone with sensory dysfunction. For example, resuming normal movement takes adjustment after riding a roller-coaster or carnival ride. Sometimes it produces a dizzy feeling or the sense that the body is still moving even when it is not. The sensory messages that the brain receives are jumbled, so the brain does not know how to tell the body to respond. The vestibular system must work to analyze the situation and relay organized information to the nervous system. The body might respond by grabbing hold of something to avoid falling over. After a few minutes the strange sensations usually subside, and the thrill from the ride is over. But during the ride and immediately after, kinesthetic awareness is greatly increased.

Learning to feel movement and developing kinesthetic awareness are important aspects of development. It is difficult to learn how to feel the difference between a contracting muscle and a stretching muscle. That may help to explain part of why children with sensory processing disorder (SPD) have difficulty with motor skills. They may sense a muscle stretching and confuse the sensation with movement. Massage increases the activity of the sensory structures, special senses, and the vestibular system, as well as kinesthetic awareness.

Adaptation

When sensory processes work correctly, people are able to feel, move, react, and interact appropriately. For example, they can pull their hand away from a hot pan on the stove, do ten jumping jacks, or take off a wool sweater because it feels itchy. However, when sensory processes do not work correctly, they might pull their hand away from a cool doorknob because it feels painful. They may have difficulty picking up a cup or pencil without looking at their hands. They might stumble while attempting to run and kick a soccer ball. In these cases something interferes with the sensory information that should be received by the brain. The lack of correct information means that a person has difficulty feeling, moving, reacting, or interacting appropriately.

In typical circumstances a person is capable of adapting to a stimulus that is not threatening or does not require a reaction. When a person becomes familiar with the surroundings or accustomed to how something feels, they no longer need to make adjustments or changes. Adaptation to stimuli is possible because the sensory receptors stop transmitting information to the brain. In children with ASD, stimuli that are not potentially threatening may be perceived as painful. Perception of a constant stimulus may be heightened because of extreme sensitivity. Therefore, the brain will continue to be aware of the stimulus. Some children may be unable to tolerate the lack of sensory input that occurs with adaptation. They will engage in movements to help provide information to the brain. When a child is unable to adapt to sensation or needs to feel stimulation, it is difficult for the brain to focus because of the confused message that is being transmitted by the sensory receptors.

Adaptation is important when understanding the sense of touch. For example, someone sits on an outdoor metal bench. He feels that the bench is cold and hard where it touches his hips and back of his legs. A typical person could choose to remain sitting until he is accustomed to the feeling of the cold, hard bench. He knows that as he sits, his body will probably warm the area of the bench underneath him. After a few moments the typical person no longer notices that the bench is hard or cold. A person with sensory processing disorder would respond differently. The cold, hard sensation from the bench might be overwhelming when he first sits down. He might immediately stand up and refuse to sit. If he remained seated, he might remain continuously aware of the unpleasant feeling of the temperature and texture of the bench under his hips and legs. Even when the bench became warm underneath him, he would still be aware that the bench was hard. This awareness of the bench would be distracting. This distraction may be so consuming that he would be unable to concentrate. His attention would focus on the bench rather than his surroundings, or events that were happening nearby. The inability to turn off the sense of touch would represent his inability to adapt to the sense of touch in a normal, everyday activity like sitting on a cold bench.

5
Touch and Communication

Compared to the other special senses, touch is unique because it serves two purposes: communication and gathering information. A person can touch or be touched by another person. Actively touching something requires a signal from the brain. Feeling something sends information to the brain. That signal tells the brain the contact is pleasant or unpleasant. Touch carries meaning.[11] Touching another person can give information about what the "toucher" feels, thinks, wants, or needs. Casual, unintentional touch may not carry meaning but it can be perceived as pleasant or unpleasant. Brushing a bare shoulder against a stranger's arm on a crowded bus is usually an unpleasant sensation. Yet casual touch, even if it is not consciously felt, can be perceived to be pleasant.[12]

Touch is a part of culture. Different types of touch are considered socially acceptable or unacceptable in various areas of the world. Often this is related to whether or not touch hurts or feels good. Slapping and hitting are forms of touch that communicate anger or frustration. They are not socially acceptable because they can cause pain or injury. Tapping is a form of touch that requests attention. In casual situations it is acceptable, but social norms sometimes dictate that touch of any sort is inappropriate. This relies on an understanding of the society and culture. Hugging is a form of touch that feels good and gives comfort. For a child with ASD, the communication and sensory functions of touch can be confused. They may not understand that various types of touch communicate different needs. A slap and a tap may serve the same purpose to them. A hug might feel like a restraint. For a non-verbal child who does not understand social cues, hitting may be a way to demand attention.

Touching someone to communicate a feeling is sort of like talking and listening at the same time. It can get that person's attention, but through the act of touching the brain is gathering information. Typical communication involves an exchange of information that is made possible by alternating talking with listening. Individuals with ASD often have difficulty developing verbal communication skills because they do not read social cues or instinctively understand relationships. These same concepts may help explain aversions to touching or being touched.

Humans instinctively gravitate toward pleasant stimuli. The stimulation can come from the body's general sense or the special senses. Stimulation can help a person learn, grow, communicate, and stay safe from harm. A stimulus can also be unpleasant and potentially dangerous. The body instinctively tries to withdraw from an unpleasant stimulus. In some situations, this is as easy as closing the eyes to filter out a bright light. Other times it is more complicated especially when the stimulus is large, involves many small stimuli, or is a single stimulus that can be perceived by one or more of the senses. An overwhelming stimulus can cause a person to act to limit the stimulus (feeling with the back of the hand instead of the palm), replace the stimulus with something more pleasant (wearing only flannel or fleece clothing), actively shift attention away from an unpleasant stimulus (scratching an insect bite), or withdraw to a position of safety (hiding in a closet).

Massage is stimulation through the sense of touch. It can be useful to help explore the tactile sense in a healthy way by exploring how different types of sensations feel. It can teach discernment and encourage kinesthetic awareness in a passive way like brushing therapy. This can broaden an ASD individual's receptiveness to different types of touch. Massage and bodywork that include joint movements and stretching can also increase proprioceptive awareness in the same way as compression of individual joints.

COMMUNICATION, SENSATION, AND MOVEMENT

In addition to talking, listening, watching, and touching, humans move to communicate. Body language includes positioning the self towards or away from another person or a stimulus as well as active movements like reaching, waving, leaning, or walking. Cognitive and social awareness are important in being able to read body language and social cues. Along with kinesthetic awareness, they are important in understanding and executing movement.

The ability to move is called motor skill.

- *Gross motor skills*, like walking, running, or jumping, use the large muscles and joints of the body.

- *Fine motor skills*, like typing, or plucking the strings of a guitar, use the small muscles and joints of the hands and fingers.

Gross movements rely on fewer nerves but more muscle fibers; fine movements use a higher ratio of nerves compared to muscle fibers. Disorders of the nervous system can affect gross or fine motor skills differently because of the number of nerves needed to produce a movement. The acquisition of motor skills occurs throughout child and adolescent development in a progressive way. Typical developmental milestones for infants begin with being able to raise the head, reach, and grasp. This progresses to walking and running in the first few years of life. These motor skills require sensory input from the body's general sense as well as the special senses. All of these motor skills are used in communication.

The line that draws communication, sensation, and movement together is circular. Movement is a form of self-expression and one of the ways humans inform others about their needs, wants, desires, and dislikes. Typically movement is purposeful; it is performed with a goal in mind. That goal may be to meet a basic survival instinct like hunger, thirst, shelter, or running from danger. It may be artistic expression through dancing or playing the piano or to seek out companionship or social interaction. Purposeful movement integrates thought (cognitive awareness), kinesthetic awareness, and proprioception into some form of self-expression within an environment. When movement is purposeful, it signals intention to other people.

A person may move just for sensory stimulation. In other words, movement is a way to seek information from the surrounding environment in a way that is either purposeful or just stimulating. A person feeling around a dark room is exploring the room while trying to avoid damage or injury. This is a sensory experience which would be purposeful. Walking across the lawn to get the newspaper is purposeful movement. Walking barefoot across the lawn would combine sensory stimulation with purposeful movement. Jumping, rocking, or spinning are sensory-seeking behaviors. The movement and the sensation provide information to the brain via the same sensory pathways stimulated by massage. They are not purposeful movement and they do not involve communication. The human brain relies on sensory input from a variety of sources. These behaviors enable the child to withdraw from the surrounding environment and any attempt at interpersonal communication. The child receives sensation but in a non-purposeful, non-interactive way.

SENSORY UNDERSTANDING

Because there are so many ways the body can receive stimulation, the brain must select which stimuli are important at any moment in time. This requires attention which is the ability to concentrate or focus on certain things while ignoring others. The ability to pay attention depends on the strength and number of the various stimuli as well as the ability to evaluate them and shift focus as needed. Athletes and theatrical or musical performers acquire this ability through their training. Divers at a swim meet must concentrate on the techniques of the upcoming dive, remember the distance between the diving platform and the pool, maintain balance as they poise to dive, and ignore the cheers, jeers, or distractions from the crowd. It is not clear whether the divers choose to consciously ignore extraneous stimuli (such as noises from the crowd) or focus so intently on the necessary sensory inputs using *selective attention* that they are no longer aware of others. Likely the inconsistencies in research on the brain indicate that attention is very individual, based on conditioning and learning.

Research on children with ASD suggests that they may have trouble focusing on a specific stimulus if they are confronted with a task that requires attention to multiple stimuli.[13–15] It is not clear whether they are unable to ignore extraneous stimuli, or have difficulty dividing attention between stimuli. The processing of stimuli using different senses occurs over different periods of time. In a typical person, sound and light are perceived faster than movement and touch.[16] In an individual with ASD, the difference in sensory processing may be due to some interference with the speed of the perception or because the timeline is disorganized.

Exposure to complex stimuli requires different avenues of sensory input as well as multiple points of attention. It can cause intense sympathetic nervous system arousal that takes the body into a state of hyper-awareness. Riding a roller-coaster or a carnival ride provides stimulation through sight, hearing, the vestibular system, and proprioception that causes sympathetic physiological arousal. Some people find the sensations associated with this kind of stimulation to be enjoyable, others do not. A person can survive this kind of stimulation for only a short time because of the intensity of the state of arousal. The intensity and variety of stimuli would likely interfere with other senses if they were exposed to a stimulus. Eating a hot dog while riding a carousel would not help a typical person taste, smell, and enjoy the hot dog because it could provide too much sensory input. The arousal caused by the perception of multiple stimuli makes the person internally aware of how they feel which makes them less aware of their surroundings and less able to interact with people around them until the stimulation ceases.

After an extreme sensory experience or a sensory overload, it takes time to return to normal. This is affected by the ability of the autonomic part of the nervous system to stimulate and inhibit the various functions that help a person rest and digest. The ability to adapt can be learned and conditioned over time. Skaters on an ice rink may feel unsteady on their feet when they leave the ice to take a break. Hockey players must learn to adapt to this sensory shift because they may enter and leave the ice rink many times during a game. Through practice and conditioning, they learn to adapt to the differences between the extreme concentration and sensory stimulus during play and the rest period. The ability to shift from sensory overload to rest probably involves a process similar to the one that enables a child to learn to fall asleep on her own. They learn to ignore sensations in favor of others by selective attention.

A child who seeks less intense stimulation like sustained pressure from a weight or a pressure vest may be using that stimulus to divert their attention from something unpleasant. It is also possible that they have differences in the sensitivity of the various mechanoreceptors. Pressure of varying intensities usually is relaxing when it is the right amount of pressure applied to a receptive area of the body. A hug from a likeable person feels good. But for that hug to be socially acceptable it should last a short time. Individuals with ASD who engage in self-stimulating behaviors are instinctively doing things to feel good. Hypo-sensitive children may crave the sensation of a roller-coaster because they feel a need for intense arousal. That need may be created by a physiological need to expend energy, to override other stimuli that they perceive as unpleasant, or the desire to avoid social interaction. Since the senses are complex and the variety for the type and magnitude of stimulation is extreme, training the senses is important for a child with a sensory processing disorder. This is especially true for the sense of touch because it contributes so much to other senses, movement, and communication.

6
How Massage and Touch Work

The sense of touch and movement of the body through stretching, joint range of motion, or exercise all involve integration of multiple systems of the body. This integration can help to train these systems to work together and more efficiently. Massage, touch, and therapeutic bodywork produce sensations in the body. These sensations follow the same pathways in the nervous system as impulses from the body's general senses and the special sense of touch. When pressure and movement are applied to muscles and joints, the brain becomes aware of the muscles and joints as well as the position of the body. The same theories that are used to explain the benefits of brushing, joint compression, and active movement also explain the benefits of massage and bodywork.

It is possible that the gate theory used to explain pain might also help to explain why massage helps a person to feel better.[17] Massage can replace an unpleasant stimulus like a muscle ache with a pleasant stimulus of pressure or rubbing. This may explain why massage and movement help to increase awareness of the body. The increased awareness can help typical clients identify when they have poor posture or are moving in an unhealthy manner. Generally massage is relaxing. When people relax, their muscles are not tense, their breathing and heart rate are lower, and they shift their attention away from external stimuli. A typical person learns how to relax by engaging in certain behaviors and finding a non-stimulating setting. An individual with ASD may not be able to pay attention to, understand, or ignore stimulus. They benefit from training of their senses. Systematic use of massage and movement can help to train kinesthetic awareness, proprioception and touch to function better. For a child with ASD or SPD, the increased awareness of the body—along with the sensory input given by massage and movement—may explain why self-stimulating behaviors decrease after massage.

Massage can also help relax tight bands of fascia that become shortened due to repetitive movements or poor posture. Tight muscles and fascia can be painful and contribute to poor posture or an altered gait. When the pain is relieved through massage, movement, or other therapeutic intervention, normal movement can be restored. Poor circulation in the body can also impair movement. Massage can help to improve circulation when it is applied in the direction of the body's circulation systems.

The various massage and bodywork styles presented in Chapters 7 to 9 use different techniques. While the techniques sometimes sound similar, there are differences in the massage styles. Sometimes the difference is in the theory behind the technique, the selection of techniques, or the context in which health is understood. The goal of massage that seems to be universal across all styles is: helping people feel better through the application of touch in a systematic manner through a client-centered approach.

PART 2

EXPLORING STYLES OF MASSAGE AND BODYWORK

7
Anatomy-Oriented Massage

The styles of massage that are reviewed in this chapter are biologically based and somatically oriented. That means they are rooted in anatomy and physiology of the body. Anatomy and physiology have been studied for decades through dissection. Massage therapists use that knowledge along with analysis of posture and movement to select techniques appropriate for their clients. Some of these modalities work on the entire body; others focus on a single area of pain or tightness. Even though the style focuses on the body, these styles of massage can have an effect on the client's psychological and emotional state.

SWEDISH MASSAGE

Swedish massage is rooted in Western (allopathic) medicine which is based on anatomy and physiology learned from dissection. It is the most common style of massage used in Western countries. Swedish massage techniques focus on muscles, tendons, ligaments, and connective tissue. The aim of Swedish massage is to improve circulation and release areas of tension. It can be effective in alleviating muscular pain. Research has frequently documented the finding that general Swedish massage promotes an overall feeling of well-being.

The origins of Swedish massage can be traced back to the turn of the nineteenth century in Europe. Per Henrick Ling developed a system of exercises known as medical gymnastics. Ling's method combined Greek and Roman medical knowledge with kung-fu-based exercises and massage techniques practiced in China. The techniques used by Ling were not original, but his systematic approach was unique. He aimed to affect different tissues in the body by performing massage strokes in a sequence. For maximum benefit, massage was a passive activity—applied to a person; the movements were intended to enhance the benefits of massage by promoting strength and flexibility. It is considered to be an early interpretation of what would eventually become the medical specialty of physical therapy.

Swedish massage is traditionally performed on a massage table with the client unclothed. The client is covered with a sheet, towel or blanket. Each part of the body is uncovered for massage and re-covered when massage to that area is completed. Massage is usually performed on bare skin using lubricant such as oil, lotion, or talc. A general Swedish massage session includes massage on the back, arms, hands, legs, feet, upper chest, abdomen, head, neck, and face. Massage to the genitals is not part of legitimate Swedish massage (and is illegal in areas where the practice of massage is regulated).

There are five basic strokes used in Swedish massage: effleurage, petrissage, friction, vibration, and tapotement.

- *Effleurage* is a gliding or rubbing stroke that is used to spread oil or lotion on the skin and warm the superficial tissues of the body. It is sometimes called rubbing and can be delivered using the palms, the side of the hand, tips of the fingers, or forearms. The length of the stroke and part of the hand or arm used depends on the area of the body being treated and the depth of pressure that is appropriate. For example, the tips of the fingers may be used to stroke the forehead, while the forearm may be used to stroke the back.

- *Petrissage* includes kneading, milking, wringing, squeezing, and compression strokes. It is used to facilitate circulation and improve range of motion of the joints by softening deeper layers of the muscles and fascia. Kneading, milking, wringing, and squeezing strokes are performed using the hands. Compression can be performed with the hand, fist, forearm, and even the elbow, knee, or foot. As with effleurage, the technique used is based on the area being treated.

- *Friction* is a technique that moves underlying fascia without gliding over the skin. It is a very small, focused stroke that is applied to the attachment sites (origin or insertion) of muscles, or to specific areas of tightness along the muscle fibers. Friction is usually performed with the fingers, thumbs, or knuckles, but may also be applied with the elbow or fist. It is used to treat specific tightness in muscle fibers and to relax muscles by releasing tension in the attachment sites of the tendons.

- *Vibration* includes several techniques that include shaking or jostling of an area as well as actual vibration and pressure of the tissue using the hands or fingers. Vibration is considered to be a stimulating stroke.

- *Tapotement* includes a variety of percussive techniques applied with fists, hands, or fingers. It is also a stimulating technique. Both vibration and tapotement aim to improve circulation.

The techniques of Swedish massage can be adapted to provide a massage treatment ranging from gentle to vigorous. Choosing from the five basic strokes, the speed and rhythm of the strokes as well as the depth of pressure can be varied to create a variety of treatments designed to meet the needs of the client. Oil or lotion is not always necessary since most of the techniques can be adapted for a client who remains clothed during the session.

Swedish massage is a unique modality, yet many other styles of massage are based on Swedish massage. The difference is often subtle. Sports, deep tissue, orthopedic, neuromuscular, and medical massage, as well as myofascial release, are all descendents of Swedish massage. These styles generally borrow some theory and technique from Swedish massage, but use other techniques in addition to the five basic Swedish massage strokes.

Research on Swedish massage has found that it improves sleep, increases attentiveness, and decreases self-stimulating behaviors in children with ASD. Even though Swedish massage is systematic, it is a very versatile modality that can be easily adapted to meet sensory needs. Some of the research protocols that used Swedish massage for ASD involved teaching parents a massage sequence. This makes the use of massage cost-efficient, and parents who have been taught to massage their child enjoyed the experience. By learning to communicate with their child through touch, parents reported that they felt closer to their child. Reports also note that children attempted to initiate the massage, indicating that they enjoyed or perceived benefit from the experience.[18–20]

SPORTS MASSAGE

The techniques that comprise sports massage are taken from a variety of other modalities. What sets sports massage apart as unique is that it aims to treat muscles used in specific sports and improve sport performance. Kneading and friction from Swedish massage, muscle stripping and traction from orthopedic massage, compression from neuromuscular massage, mobilization from deep tissue massage, along with targeted stretching are among the techniques used by a sports massage therapist.

The origins of sports massage are unclear, but it likely arose from medical gymnastics and Swedish massage used for athletes. Various types of "rubdowns" and stretching have been given to athletes for centuries. It began to receive widespread attention in the early twentieth century as a possible tool to help improve athletic performance. In the mid-1980s it became recognized as a massage specialty.

Sports massage does not generally address the entire body. Rather the focus is on muscles that are involved in the skills used in the chosen sport, like running, jumping, hitting, catching, and throwing. The repetition of these movements in sport along with the total body training necessary to be competitive often leave athletes achy, tired, or sore. During sports massage, which is usually performed on a massage table, the client may wear loose clothing or be unclothed and covered with a sheet or towel. Oil or lotion is sometimes used in sports massage, but is not always necessary.

Assessment of the athlete's posture and movements are used to aid the massage therapist in understanding where muscle imbalances (in strength and length) occur. When muscles needed for movements are weak, the athlete can compensate by moving the body in an unnatural manner. When overused muscles are chronically tight, it also affects the ability of the athlete to move naturally. In either case, the athlete's performance is adversely affected.

Athletic training and competition involves periodization. This involves scheduling specific training activities to help achieve optimal performance. An athlete's training regimen involves general training for fitness and skills, preparation for competition, the event or competitive season, a post-event or post-season recovery. Sports massage is adapted to aid the athlete during different phases of training and recovery.

Massage is used before an event to prepare the muscles for competition (*pre-event*) and after an event to aid in cooling down (*post-event*). In sports massage, techniques are selected based on their ability to improve circulation, stimulate, relax, or lengthen specific muscles. Rapid, deep kneading, jostling of the joints, and quick range-of-motion movements are used pre-event to prepare the body for activity. Slow strokes, rocking motions, and gentle stretches are used to loosen muscles and soften connective tissues in post-event massage. Management of muscle cramping in post-event massage is important. Compression, stretching, or a combination of both can be used to alleviate cramps. Sports massage involves a delicate balance between relaxing muscles and connective tissues while enabling athletes to use those muscles in their sport. The timing of the massage treatment and adapting of the techniques is important to promote performance.

For example, pre-event sports massage for baseball pitchers would focus on the chest, shoulder, upper back, arm, and hand on their pitching side. Immediately before a practice or game, vigorous movements such as compression, kneading, and jostling would aim to warm up these areas. Encouraging the pitcher to walk and stretch the legs, hips, lower back, and torso would also be useful because the movement of pitching involves the leg and hip opposite the pitching arm as well as the torso. A post-event sports massage for the pitcher should take place within a few hours after the event. It would involve the whole body (chest, shoulder, upper back, arm, and hand on the pitching side as well as the legs, hips, lower back, and torso). The techniques would include moderate kneading, gentle compressions, and slow stretching. Pre-event massage usually involves moderate to deep pressure; post-event massage usually involves moderate pressure. In the case of chronic pain or injury, cryotherapy would be used post-event to alleviate potential inflammation.

Ongoing massage treatments (*maintenance*) can help to alleviate muscle imbalances brought on by repetitive movements used in sports. Massage techniques are often used in rehabilitation of minor injuries including sprains, strains, stress fractures, and inflammatory conditions related to overuse. Application of heat (*thermotherapy*) and cold (*cryotherapy*) are also used in sports massage. Thermotherapy is used to warm up muscles before events; cryotherapy is used after events to reduce potential inflammation due to minor injury or overuse. Alternating hot and cold therapies (contrast bathing) is often recommended in maintenance sports massage to facilitate healing of chronic injuries.

Stretching is an important aspect of athletic performance and sports massage. Joints need flexibility and muscles that act on joints need balance to maintain proper posture and movement. Stretching extends the length of a muscle or group of muscles that move a joint. A stretch lengthens not only the fibers of a muscle, but also the tendons and fascia that enclose the muscle fibers. Stretching can release chronically shortened muscles due to activities (like sports) or habits (like poor posture).

Sports massage uses stretching techniques to improve muscle function and proprioceptive awareness. There are different sensory receptors in tendons and ligaments. Stretching activities target the muscle fibers and fascia that are located outside of joints. Therefore, stretching has an indirect affect on proprioception which is important for individuals with sensory integration disorders. Ligaments are non-contractile tissue that connect bones together to form a joint. Ligaments can stretch but may not necessarily relax. Ligaments should not be stretched because joints need the ligaments to maintain stability.

Stretches can be active or passive.

- *Active stretching* is when the client moves the target joint or stretches the joint without assistance from a practitioner or stretching device.

- *Passive stretching* is when the joint is relaxed during the stretch; usually this stretch is performed by a practitioner while the client is relaxed or by the client using a stretching assistive device such as a strap, weight, or bar.

Stretching the knees to the chest can be performed passively (see Figure 7.1) when the practitioner applies the stretch, or actively if clients pull their own knees to the chest.

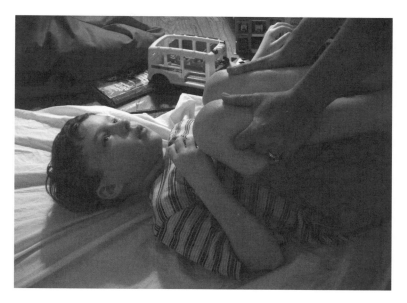

Figure 7.1 Sports massage

Both active and passive stretches can be performed in a static or dynamic manner.

- *Static stretching* is customarily held for 10–30 seconds to allow the target muscle(s) to relax.

- *Dynamic stretching* uses movement and momentum to stretch a joint to its full range of motion.

- *Ballistic stretching* is a type of dynamic stretching that uses bouncing movements to extend the joint beyond its range of motion. Ballistic stretches involve more movement with the end range of the stretch being held for only 1–3 seconds. Static, dynamic, and ballistic stretches can be active or passively performed.

Muscles work in opposition. A muscle cannot contract and be stretched at the same time. So when a muscle (agonist) contracts, its opponent (antagonist) is relaxed. This is called *reciprocal inhibition.* These techniques may be used in physical therapy and exercise physiology, as well as massage. Following are descriptions of three stretching techniques that use this theory.

- *Proprioceptive Neuromuscular Facilitation* (PNF) is a type of stretching that employs the theory of reciprocal inhibition by using sequenced patterns of muscle contraction and stretching. There are several different patterns of muscle activation used in PNF sequences.

- *Active Isolated Stretching* (AIS) uses PNF techniques along with myofascial release techniques to stretch an isolated movement of a joint. The client contracts (the agonist) for a few seconds then the practitioner stretches the antagonist muscle for a few seconds. After a rest phase, the sequence is repeated.

- *Muscle Energy Technique* (MET) uses isometric muscle contractions followed by a relaxation phase. The practitioner directs the client and applies resistance against the contraction to encourage the stretch. The criteria for selecting muscles and the length of time that muscles contract and relax vary according to different approaches. When resistance is applied during muscle contractions, it helps train muscles to contract properly.

All these styles of stretching require participation by the client. They can significantly increase range of motion because they are deep stretching techniques that aim to improve range of motion in a specific area of the body. This happens through release of tight muscles, tendons, connective tissues, and fascia.

Range of motion is passive or active movement of a joint without bringing a muscle into a stretch. It usually involves slow, continuous movement. In sports massage, range of motion is used to increase awareness of movement. It is also used in medical massage for individuals who are unable to voluntarily move.

The pacing and depth of most types of stretches can be adapted to warmup muscles before or cool down after an activity or sports event. While research has not evaluated the benefits of sports massage for ASD, the selection and adaptation of massage techniques offers a useful model. There is research evidence from the field of exercise physiology that stretching can prevent injury in athletes by helping the body to warm up prior to activity and cool down after activity. The concepts used in pre- and post-event massage are based on warm-up and cool-down theories from sport performance and exercise physiology. Pre-event massage techniques and concepts are suitable for children who are non-responsive to touch (hypo-sensitive). The techniques and concepts of post-event massage are suitable for children who are extremely sensitive to touch (hyper-sensitive) or need encouragement to become receptive to touch.

A very useful application of sports massage for ASD involves techniques used on leg muscles of runners and sprinters. Often these athletes have tight muscles along the posterior upper and lower legs. These muscles (hamstrings, gastrocnemius, and soleus) are also frequently tight in children with ASD who "toe-walk." Massage and stretching techniques similar to those used in maintenance massage for athletes can be used on the children to lengthen these shortened muscles. These are strong muscles that can become very tight over time. The approach for children should be gentle at first. Non-verbal children should be observed for feedback about pain threshold.

Sports massage may also be helpful for children who have poor motor skills. Analysis of movement can help the massage therapist to identify muscles or muscle groups that are not activating properly. This is similar to analysis done for baseball pitchers, golfers, and tennis players. Movement restrictions that are due to tight muscles can be effectively targeted with sports massage.

Sometimes the terms *deep tissue, sports massage, neuromuscular, medical,* and *orthopedic massage* are used interchangeably. But different practitioners and instructors identify the differences in the goals, approaches, and expected outcomes of massage treatment. They share similar theories and techniques. All of these types of massage focus on detailed massage of muscles to facilitate joint movement.

DEEP TISSUE MASSAGE

Deep tissue massage is not a single style of massage. Rather it is an integration of techniques that aim to lengthen habitually shortened muscles and connective tissue or release areas of extremely tight fascia. Restrictions in the muscles, fascia, and soft tissue can contribute to muscle imbalances around the joints causing pain and altered movement. Deep tissue massage uses techniques from Swedish massage, neuromuscular massage, myofascial release, and stretching.

Deep tissue massage is a fairly recent development in massage that likely originated during the resurgence in massage in Western countries during the mid-twentieth century. The exact beginnings of deep tissue massage are not known. It is possible that it grew organically out of Swedish massage when massage clients requested deeper pressure during the massage. It has come to be identified as a specialty in the massage and bodywork field. The term "deep" is used alternatively to refer to long-term chronic pain or to massage that addresses muscles and fascia that lie deep within the body.

A common misconception about deep tissue massage is that it is painful. It is not unusual for a client to be somewhat sore after the massage because of the release in the tight tissues.

Deep tissue massage is not forceful. The amount of pressure may be firm, but should not aim to cause bruising or injury. Softer pressure along with movement of a joint (mobilization) is used to release soft tissue. Deep tissue practitioners speak of working on the body in "layers." They are referring to release of the muscles and fascia closest to the surface of the body before trying to access the muscles and fascia that lie deeper within.

A deep tissue massage session focuses on a target area of chronic pain, tension, or muscle imbalance. It may be part of a general massage session, or an entire massage to one area of the body. Deep tissue massage is usually performed on a massage table with the client unclothed and covered with a sheet or towel. If oil or lotion is used, it is used sparingly so that the massage therapist can have better traction on the skin.

Massage therapists generally conduct a pre-massage assessment. They may interview the client about occupation, daily habits, and recreational activities. They may ask the client whether pain in the targeted area occurs or gets better with particular movements. The massage therapist may also observe the client's posture for possible signs of muscular imbalance.

For example, a client suffers from chronic shoulder pain. She reveals that she works on a computer, walks her dog several times each day, and plays tennis regularly. The client sometimes feels pain in her neck when she sits for too long or when she pulls a shirt on over her head. She reports that she has tried relaxation massage and stretching, but still feels pain and tension on a daily basis. Assessment of her posture reveals that her shoulders hunch forward and her arms rotate inward, when she stands. This assessment indicates that several muscles are tight (pectoralis major, latissimus dorsi, and subscapularis) compared to the other muscles around her shoulder and neck. Based on this assessment, the massage therapist focuses the session on these specific muscles of the client's back, neck, chest, and shoulders. He chooses techniques to release tight muscle fibers and fascia in these areas.

Deep tissue massage has not been evaluated for ASDs. As with a typical population, it may be useful for individuals who have muscle imbalances or report chronic musculoskeletal pain. Possible applications for deep tissue are for shortened calf muscles due to toe-walking. Massage application would be similar to sports massage approach. Deep tissue may also be useful to provide deep stimulation for children who flap their hands. While brushing is routinely recommended in sensory therapy for the hands and forearms, it can irritate sensitive skin. Deep tissue massage may be able to serve a similar function without irritation by stimulating sensory receptors on the skin as well as deep within the tissues.

ORTHOPEDIC MASSAGE

Orthopedic massage is use of massage techniques to treat musculoskeletal pain and to aid in rehabilitation of injuries. Like sports massage and deep tissue massage, orthopedic massage is rooted in focus rather than a specific technical approach. The focus of orthopedic massage is on the muscles involved in movement as well as postural muscles that align the body. Called musculoskeletal disorders, the conditions treated by orthopedic massage are in various stages of rehabilitation—ranging from acute to long-term conditions. Orthopedic massage relies on the skill of the massage therapist who is trained to use a variety of techniques. The techniques used in orthopedic massage are taken from Swedish massage, neuromuscular massage, myofascial release, stretching, and lymphatic drainage. Sometimes a deep tissue approach is needed to facilitate change in chronically tightened muscles and fascia.

Orthopedic massage owes its origins to the rise of chiropractic and osteopathic medicine in the late nineteenth century as well as the conventional medical specialty of orthopedics, and physical therapy. All of these healthcare specialties aim to treat and rehabilitate some aspect of injury to the musculoskeletal system. The actual beginnings of orthopedic massage are very recent—the late twentieth century. Around this time, the field of massage therapy was immersed in becoming more professional with the development of standards for education and practice, professional associations, certifications and licensure. Education in anatomy, physiology, and kinesiology became a standardized part of massage training. Now, as well as then, massage therapists are taught to evaluate muscle strength and range of motion, and posture as well as assess normal patterns of gait (locomotion) and joint movement. This training provides the foundation to enable the massage therapist to target the massage towards specific muscles that interfere with normal movement. Often a massage therapist specializing in orthopedic massage may be found working with a chiropractor, in a sports or injury rehabilitation center, as well as in private practice.

Orthopedic massage is generally performed with the client lying on a massage table. Depending on the area of the body in need of attention, the client may remain clothed or partially clothed during the session. Oil or lotion may be used depending on the need for lubrication in the techniques the massage therapist uses in the massage. For some conditions orthopedic massage sessions are short and frequent (twenty minutes, twice per week). For other conditions, the sessions may be longer and less frequent (one hour every week). Generally, orthopedic massage involves a series of massage sessions to allow the targeted muscles and fascia time to adapt to the treatment.

Often a client who seeks orthopedic massage will have a medical diagnosis for a musculoskeletal disorder and may have received medical treatment. The massage therapist will still perform assessment of the affected area to better understand what muscles are affected and which techniques are most appropriate. Based on the medical diagnosis and the assessment, the massage therapist designs a treatment. The session is created to use the most appropriate techniques to alleviate pain, reduce inflammation, lengthen contracted muscles, and restore optimal movement.

Massage therapists trained in orthopedic massage follow protocols for specific disorders. An example of orthopedic massage would be a client who suffers from sciatica. He reports pain that shoots down his leg. This condition has occurred on and off for several years. Despite receiving a variety of treatments, the pain has returned. A pre-massage assessment would evaluate specific muscles in the back of his hip (the piriformis, other lateral rotators of the hip), and the back of his leg (the hamstring muscle group). This assessment would involve normal range of motion of his hips, the strength of these muscles, as well as the ability of his hip and low back to stretch. The massage therapist would also observe the client's posture. Based on the results of this assessment, the massage therapist would design a massage treatment that focused on the client's low back, hip, thigh, and leg.

The effect of orthopedic massage for ASD has not been evaluated. Like deep tissue and sports massage, an orthopedic approach may be appropriate for individuals who have muscle imbalances or chronic musculoskeletal pain. The approach for toe-walking would be similar to that used in sports massage or deep tissue massage. The focus of orthopedic massage on locomotion makes it a promising potential therapy for children with ASD who have difficulty with gross motor skills. Comprehensive postural assessment may reveal patterns of muscle weakness or contracture that interfere with normal movement. Regular, focused massage may help to restore movement and improve gross motor skills.

NEUROMUSCULAR MASSAGE

Neuromuscular massage is a local application of massage techniques that aim to treat chronic pain and soft tissue injury in local areas of the body. Often referred to as neuromuscular therapy (NMT) it focuses on releasing nerve impingement, treating myofascial trigger points, and correcting muscle imbalances. There are many different styles of neuromuscular massage, some of which are trademarked. They arise from two basic theoretical approaches to neuromuscular massage: the European approach and the American approach. These two approaches came into existence in Europe and the United States in the same time period.

The European version grew out of chiropractic and naturopathic medicine and focused on manipulation of muscles and joints to restore posture and normal movement. The American version arose from conventional medicine and focused on myofascial trigger points. These hyper-sensitive spots in muscles occur because of an injury in that area. The injury creates a nodule in the muscle and fascia that restricts circulation. This becomes a problem that interferes with posture and normal movement. Pressing on the nodules causes predictable patterns of referred pain (pain that is felt a distance away from the actual myofascial trigger point). The focus of American neuromuscular massage is to alleviate pain by releasing the myofascial trigger point. Dr. Janet G. Travell was President John F. Kennedy's personal physician and a pioneer in the area of myofascial trigger points. She treated President Kennedy for chronic back pain.

Some of the techniques used in European neuromuscular massage are referred to as *manipulation*. But these are different than chiropractic adjustments or orthopedic manipulation, because the techniques focus only on the soft tissues (muscles, tendons, and fascia) rather than adjustments or alignment of bones. Thumb and finger stroking, skin rolling, pressure, percussion, Muscle Energy Techniques, and Proprioceptive Neuromuscular Facilitation are techniques used in European neuromuscular massage. American neuromuscular massage uses sustained pressure directly on trigger points. This pressure can be applied with fingers, hands, or elbows as well as massage tools specially made for this purpose. The pressure may be combined with movement or deep stretching of the target muscle may be performed after the trigger point releases. Often one muscle will have several trigger points. Locating and treating all of the trigger points is necessary for pain relief. Thermotherapy (heat) and cryotherapy (cold) are used in European and American neuromuscular massage.

Neuromuscular massage is versatile. It can be performed with the client lying on a massage table. Depending on the area of the body being treated, the client may remain fully or partially clothed, or be unclothed and covered with a sheet or towel. Neuromuscular techniques can also be used in chair massage. A series of short sessions focusing the massage on the injured area can be very effective in rehabilitation. The techniques can also be integrated into a Swedish, sports, or orthopedic massage session when they are appropriate in the massage treatment plan.

European and American neuromuscular massage share the same goal: to restore muscle balance and alignment of the body by releasing tightness and improving circulation in specific muscles. Therefore, the massage therapist will often perform extensive assessment of the area of the body that will be treated. Specific stretching exercises or regular use of heat or cold packs are frequently recommended by the massage therapist.

There are no studies to date that evaluate the use of neuromuscular massage for ASDs. It may be helpful for any child with ASD who suffers from chronic pain due to a muscle injury, has trigger points, or posture problems. Like orthopedic massage, deep tissue, and sports massage, some of the techniques may be useful to release tightness in the calf muscles that can occur with toe-walking. Deep, targeted pressure to the forearms and hands may help to provide sensory input for children who engage in hand-flapping or other self-stimulating behaviors with the arms and hands.

MYOFASCIAL RELEASE

Myofascial release is a concept of massage that aims to restore posture and movement by stretching tight bands of fascia in the muscles and skin. There are several different approaches to myofascial release with names that involve variations on combinations of words like "myo," "fascia," "connective tissue," "massage," and "release." *Myo* means muscle and *fascia* means tissue. The various types of myofascial release share a common goal: to release tightness in muscles by extending fascia—the tissue that surrounds muscle.

Muscle tightness occurs because the contractile muscle fibers lose their extensibility. That means that after they shorten to produce movement, they no longer return to the appropriate resting length. Over time this can affect the alignment of joints. When one muscle is tight, the muscle that performs the opposite action can become weak. For example, a person who works at a computer all day may acquire a hunched posture due to tightness in the muscles of the chest and front of the shoulders. Over time, the upper back muscles and muscles of the back of the shoulders may become weaker. This makes the posture worse because they lack strength in the back muscles as well as the ability to stretch or lengthen the front muscles.

One of the factors that affects posture and joint alignment when a person's muscles are tight is the fascia. The tight muscle pulls the bones of the joint in one direction. When the opposite muscle tries to contract, it may not be capable of adequate strength to pull the bones in the other direction. Muscles can be stimulated by motor neurons to relax. Fascia does not respond to stimulation. If it tightens or shortens, it must be gently lengthened. Much in the same way a knit sweater can be reshaped after it has been washed, myofascial release applies tension in different directions to lengthen fascia.

The origins of myofascial release lie within osteopathic medicine. Myofascial techniques were used by osteopaths in the United States during the late nineteenth century. The term myofascial release came into vogue in the 1960s. Variations of myofascial release are now used by osteopaths, physical therapists, and massage therapists.

Myofascial release works on specific areas of the body using the hands, fingers, forearms, or fists. It is performed slowly to allow the muscles to relax so the fascia can soften and release. Techniques include skin rolling, stroking, stretches, compression, release, and traction techniques. This style of massage is not forceful, but can often be felt deep within the body when tight fascia relaxes.

Myofascial release is usually performed with the client lying on a massage table. The techniques may also be integrated into a full-body Swedish, orthopedic, deep tissue, or sports massage session or used alone in a session that focuses on a specific problem area. Myofascial release practitioners conduct a thorough assessment of posture, observe movement, and feel the soft tissue in the affected area (*palpation*). Oil and lotion are not used in myofascial release. This helps the practitioner get traction on the skin and feel the target area release.

Specific techniques are chosen depending on the muscles and joints that will be targeted in the session. For muscles the release may follow the direction of muscle action, or it may be performed across the muscle. This depends on where the tightness occurs in the muscle. Tightness in joints may be due to tight tissue in the muscle, tendon, or the joint capsule. In joints, the release follows the direction of a natural joint movement. The joints of the body are structured to allow movement in specific directions (*planes*). Stretching in these planes or in the perpendicular direction can release tight fascia. Figure 7.2 shows a myofascial release technique on the calf muscles.

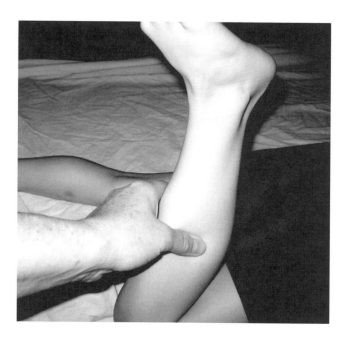

Figure 7.2 Myofascial release

Myofascial release has not yet been evaluated for clients with ASD. Like sports, deep tissue, neuromuscular, and orthopedic massage, it may help restore alignment to the lower leg muscles in children who "toe-walk." For children who respond to compression therapy, holding, and squeezing myofascial release may be useful to increase sensory awareness because it can target joints as well as layers of soft tissues. One difficulty with myofascial release is that young children often do not stay still during massage treatment. Care should be taken to maintain alignment when releasing or tractioning the joints.

MEDICAL MASSAGE

Medical massage can be described as the use of massage to treat medical conditions that have been diagnosed by a primary healthcare provider. This includes any pathological condition that occurs anywhere in the body. Medical massage is a theoretical approach rather than specific techniques.

The first references to the use of massage for medical conditions in English-language medical journals appeared in the late nineteenth century. Massage was used to treat constipation, migraines, and skin conditions as well as musculoskeletal problems. There are also reports of massage being a vital part of rehabilitation for soldiers wounded in World War I. Despite extensive use of massage in medicine, it evolved into an alternative therapy with the professionalization of conventional medical education in the early twentieth century. The Flexner Report, published in 1910, was a critical evaluation of medical education in the United States. This led to standardization of admissions requirements and development of curriculum rooted in the biological sciences. Holistic and natural therapies—like massage—were dropped from conventional medical education.

Massage has traditionally served two basic purposes in healthcare. It has been used for wellness and relaxation or it has been employed to alleviate signs or symptoms of a disease or disorder. For some clients, massage initially becomes part of their healthcare routine because of an illness, pathological disorder, or medical condition. They may then transition to using massage for wellness; as part of their self-care regimen. The approach and application of medical massage is what makes it unique. Pediatric medical massage is any type of massage that is used with the goal of alleviating the signs or symptoms of a medical condition for an infant or child.

A medical massage therapist often has an arsenal of techniques borrowed from Swedish massage and related modalities. Massage therapists who practice medical massage receive training in pathophysiology (the study of diseases), anatomy, physiology, and kinesiology. They combine this knowledge with their massage training to choose the best approach to treat the client. In some cases massage can be an effective complementary therapy to alleviate symptoms of the condition. In other cases, it may not alter the course of a disease or disorder, but can help the client feel better by helping them relax.

There are several massage techniques that fall within the category of medical massage as an integrative therapy.

- *Ocular massage* is used to release blockage in tear ducts of infants.

- *Perineal massage* can relax pelvic muscles in preparation for childbirth.

- *Prostatic massage* is used to improve prostate gland function.

These are all applications of medical massage that are integrated with conventional medicine and performed by medical personnel rather than massage therapists. When parental massage is also used to encourage weight gain in premature infants, alleviate constipation, or release blocked tear ducts, it is considered pediatric medical massage. These approaches would aid in bonding, but the goal of the treatment would be to address a medical condition.

One massage modality that is used for medical purposes is *lymphatic drainage*. This approach uses light pressure in a systematic manner that follows the direction of the circulation of lymph and blood in areas of the body where there is inflammation due to injury or disease. Lymphatic drainage is used to treat conditions like sprained ankles as well as inflammation that can occur as a result of surgery for breast cancer.

Medical massage can be performed wherever the client is comfortable: massage table, massage chair, hospital bed, wheelchair, lounge chair, or the client's own bed at home. Some hospitals let nurses trained in massage work with patients to help alleviate anxiety. The client may remain fully or partly clothed during the massage, which can last anywhere from a few minutes to a full one-hour session. The length of the session and massage treatment protocol depends on the client's needs, expectations, and medical condition. Additionally, the use of oil or lotion depends on the area of the body being treated, the techniques used in the massage, as well as the medical condition of the client.

Any use of massage to treat sensory or muscle problems associated with ASD would be considered medical massage, regardless of the techniques and treatment protocol used. As noted elsewhere in this book, research has found that individuals with ASD can benefit from massage. A variety of research studies have found that massage has a favorable affect on a variety of diseases and disorders. A few of the physical benefits of medical massage include: growth in premature infants, decreased pain in fibromyalgia, and reduced spasticity in multiple sclerosis. The psychological benefits of medical massage have found improvements in measures of stress and anxiety in cancer patients, burn victims, and end-stage renal patients. This is important because stress and anxiety can increase susceptibility to disease and some disorders and exacerbate existing symptoms. Across all of these studies (and much more research), different techniques and treatment designs have been used. What the studies have in common is that the conditions benefited from the use of massage as a complementary therapy.

CRANIOSACRAL THERAPY

Craniosacral therapy uses very gentle touch that is focused on the head and spine. Sometimes called cranialsacral therapy, it aims to promote the flow of fluid within the central nervous system by eliminating restrictions caused by tissues and bones that surround the fluid. In craniosacral therapy gentle manipulations are performed to the bones, skin, and tissues that protect the central nervous system. These manipulations release blockages of cerebrospinal fluid.

Craniosacral therapy arose from osteopathic medicine in the early twentieth century. A prevailing anatomical theory at that time (and still today) was that the bones of the skull became fused during normal development. Once fused, they were no longer capable of movement. An osteopath, William Sutherland, believed that the bones could continue to move. Thus they could be manipulated. Another osteopath, John Upledger, reported feeling a pulse in the head and spinal cord that was different than the pulse of the heart. Dr. Upledger focused his work on feeling the pulse of the fluid of the central nervous system—cerebrospinal fluid. He believed that tightness in the fascia of the central nervous system or improper position of the bones could restrict the flow of cerebrospinal fluid.

The term *cranium* refers to the head or skull. The term *sacrum* refers to a large bone at the base of the spine that forms part of the pelvis. Together with the vertebrae of the spine, the cranial bones and the sacrum enclose the brain and spinal cord. Thus, the cranial bones and the sacrum protect the opposite ends of the central nervous system. As noted in Chapter 3, the central nervous system is responsible for receiving and understanding information and acting on it when necessary.

Several layers of fascia (membranes or *meninges*) cover the brain and spinal cord. This fascia separates the brain into different compartments (*ventricles*) and encloses the spinal cord. Cerebrospinal fluid is a clear substance which circulates between the layers of fascia and between the fascia and the bones. Essentially, the brain and spinal cord float in cerebrospinal fluid, that is encapsulated in layers of membranes, which are protected by the skull, the bones of the vertebral column, and the sacrum. The functions of cerebrospinal fluid are to protect, nourish, and remove wastes from the brain and spinal cord. It is also thought to play a role in communication within the central nervous system.

The skull is made up of twenty-two bones. Fourteen of these bones form the structure of the face and jaw. Eight bones form the cranium which is the covering for the brain. During typical growth and development, the eight bones of the cranium fuse together to form a continuous protective shell around the brain. Thirteen of the bones of the face also fuse together. Conventional anatomy and physiology teaches that the jaw is the only part of the skull that is moveable. Craniosacral therapy practitioners believe that there is a slight movement of the cranial bones that occurs with the circulation of cerebrospinal fluid. This movement can be observed by carefully feeling with the hands. Craniosacral therapy aims to promote the natural rhythmic circulation of cerebrospinal fluid by locating and releasing restrictions within the fluid or caused by the membranes or bones.

A craniosacral therapy session is performed with the client fully clothed lying on a massage table. Standard sessions last one hour, but a treatment can be as short as fifteen or twenty minutes. The practitioner feels different areas of the head and spine to evaluate the pulse of cerebrospinal fluid. The practitioner may also touch other areas of the body for restrictions in fascia. The rhythms of circulation in the body can be observed in the cardiovascular system by feeling the pulse and in the respiratory system by feeling or observing movement of the ribcage. Practitioners of craniosacral therapy observe the flow of cerebrospinal fluid by "listening" through touch. Just as blood circulates through the body in a rhythm, cerebrospinal fluid has a unique rhythm. By palpating or holding the skull (see Figure 7.3) or the sacrum, the craniosacral practitioner feels movement of the bones in response to the flow of cerebrospinal fluid. Once variations in cerebrospinal fluid rhythm are established, gentle pressure (the weight of a nickel) is used to interrupt and restart the flow of cerebrospinal fluid. Craniosacral therapy practitioners may also evaluate the fascia of the body for tightness and/ or gently manipulate the bones of the skull, spine, or sacrum. Stretches and movement may be used to release tension in the spine or neck. Craniosacral therapy is sometimes described as a somato-emotional experience. Release of tension in the fascia often affects clients on an emotional level.

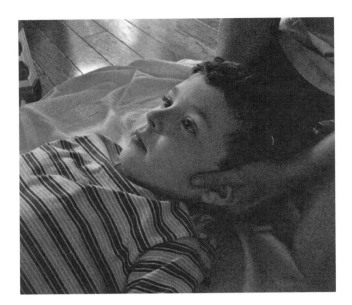

Figure 7.3 Craniosacral therapy

Several different theories are presented regarding ASD within the context of craniosacral therapy. Neurological differences in the brain have been found in high-functioning individuals with autism.[21] Craniosacral practitioners believe that cerebrospinal fluid must flow correctly to promote brain function. Craniosacral practitioners believe that ASD is related to restrictions in the membranes that surround the cerebrospinal fluid. This causes compression in the low back or in the bones of the skull (at the level of the ears). Craniosacral therapy aims to alleviate restrictions and compression and restore health to the central nervous system of individuals with ASD. There are anecdotal reports that craniosacral therapy reduced self-stimulating behaviors in children with ASD.[22] These reports are similar to the findings from studies evaluating the use of other massage modalities for ASD. However, there is little actual research evidence supporting the use of craniosacral therapy for ASD. The potential benefits are rooted in the theory that craniosacral therapy can restore flow of cerebrospinal fluid to the specific areas of the brain (motor cortex, sensory cortex, as well as the areas of the brain responsible for language, the special senses, and coordination) that may not function properly in a child with ASD.

The light touch used in craniosacral therapy may be beneficial for children who are hyper-sensitive to touch. However, light touch may be inappropriate and irritating for hypo-sensitive children. Craniosacral therapy is generally practiced with the client lying very still. That may be difficult for children who seek stimulation through movement.

STRUCTURAL INTEGRATION

Structural Integration is a distinct form of connective tissue work that aims to restore optimal alignment of the body. It was developed in the middle of the twentieth century by Ida Rolf, a biochemist by training. Dr. Rolf taught yoga and sampled a variety of alternative therapies including chiropractic and osteopathy. Structural Integration—also known as Rolfing— grew out of her interest in movement and restoring alignment to the body.

Rolf's studies led her to the conclusion that the key to proper alignment of the skeleton could be found in the connective tissues and fascia. She envisioned the fascia as a layer of mesh that was continuous throughout the body. Unlike most forms of massage that focus on muscles as well as fascia, Structural Integration addresses only the fascial system.

Although it is a form of therapeutic massage, Structural Integration is usually referred to as "bodywork." Like many other forms of massage and bodywork, there are different approaches to Structural Integration. All Structural Integration variations have the same goal: to release fascia and connective tissue from nearby muscles and other connective tissue.

Connections between different areas of the body through this network of fascia mean that tight fascia in one area can cause problems with movement in another area. For example, pain in the right knee might contribute to tightness in the left hip or right shoulder because the body compensates movement to accommodate the right knee.

Structural Integration begins with a series of ten sessions that target the body in different sections. The sessions are designed to be performed in sequence. Maintenance sessions may be useful to help clients remain free of fascial restrictions. A key component of Structural Integration is evaluation of the client's posture and movement. The practitioner then uses a variety of techniques on the targeted areas of the body including light or deep pressure, stretching, and joint mobilization to release tight fascia. Although the approach is systematic, the types of touch used in the sessions are individual for each practitioner. Practitioners may use their hands, fingers, arms, elbows, or fists depending on the area of the body and the tightness they feel in the fascia. The client may remain partly clothed during the session. Structural Integration sessions are performed with the client lying or sitting on a massage table or standing. The position depends on the section of the body being treated in that session.

Structural Integration is not forceful, but the release of tight connective tissue can be painful and powerful for some clients. The goal is to release the tissue in stages (from surface to deep within the body) and promote better posture and movement habits. Practitioners may recommend stretching programs to help maintain the benefits of the bodywork. Some Structural Integration clients have reported emotional releases in response to the release of certain restricted areas in the body. Many clients report that they feel transformed after the series of ten sessions.

Research has found that Structural Integration can aid in correcting chronic problems with posture and movement. In that way, it may improve performance in athletes, dancers, and others who use their body for work or artistic expression. It has not been systematically evaluated for children with ASD. There are anecdotal reports that children with ASD responded favorably to Structural Integration sessions. Children with ASD who have postural problems may benefit from Structural Integration. It is conceivable that the deep release of connective tissue may meet a sensory need for some individuals with ASD.

8 Energy-Based Bodywork

Energy-based bodywork takes a metaphysical approach to health and well-being. A common theme among different styles is that there is a network of energy that connects every aspect of life. That includes physical functions, thoughts, emotions and interactions between different people, as well as people and the surrounding environment. When a person has an energetic imbalance, it can affect their physical function but it also interferes with their psychological and emotional well-being. The connection between mind, body, and spirit is important in energy-based massage and bodywork.

The National Center for Complementary and Alternative Medicine (NCCAM) refers to energy-based massage and bodywork as part of biofield therapies. These healing techniques rely on the movement or manipulation of some type of energy. The recognition that energy is felt rather than seen is an essential feature of biofield healing. The practitioner's intuition and ability to sense or feel energy is vital to the healing practices. The philosophical and cultural interpretations of energy and touch are expressed in many different ways around the world. The words used to describe energy, the specific areas where energy is located, and the direction of energy flow is explained and understood differently. Some of these styles are considered non-contact because they do not involve manipulation through actual touch techniques. The non-contact approaches rely heavily on visualization and perception of energy. Although non-contact massage is not *actually* massage or bodywork, it does involve treatment that is applied to the body.

Some styles of energy healing are related to the tradition of "laying on of the hands" practices. This approach can be found in folk healing, traditional medicine, spiritual and religious interactions and the new age movement. The energy-based massage arena includes recently developed styles as well as traditional forms of bodywork that have been in existence for thousands of years. Some forms of energy-based massage blend theories and techniques from knowledge of anatomy and physiology, psychology, and Eastern forms of traditional medicine. Traditional medical systems in Asia often included massage or bodywork along with nutritional therapies, herbal remedies, and spiritual healing. A common goal of energy-based bodywork is to rebalance energy. Disease or illness occurs when energy is out of balance. Various assessment methods may be used to identify areas of weak or excess energy. Treatment aims to smooth energy into an even flow.

The terms *bio-energetic* and *somato-energetic* are sometimes used to describe newly developed massage styles that aim to treat physical conditions through touch or manipulation of energy. The intention behind the treatment is important. Different types of touch may be used and various areas of the body may be touched that are often quite distant from the sign or symptom. For example, touch to the feet or legs can be used to alleviate headache pain. Some energy therapies are non-contact approaches to energy healing because they do not involve touch. These therapies would not likely have any direct sensory benefit for an individual with ASD. Since the sensory receptors of the nervous system are not directly stimulated, there would not be a response. However, it is important to note that the non-contact therapies are not inherently harmful. Clients who receive these therapies may feel better because they are aware of the practitioner's intent to help them heal. For clients who have pain or other symptoms of illness, energy therapies may simply shift the focus of their attention away from the pain or symptom. Practitioners perceive a benefit because they are trying to help someone feel better. For caregivers this can be an important step toward self-care.

Most forms of energy-based massage and bodywork are considered holistic because they acknowledge the connection between physical health and emotional or psychological traits. The practitioner of an energy-based therapy is often viewed as a facilitator that helps the client heal his or her own body. In this way the client is often considered a partner in the healing process. The following text will introduce modalities that address the energetic fields in and around the body.

REFLEXOLOGY

Reflexology is pressure and massage of specific zones on the hands and feet. These zones correspond to different organs and areas of the body. Pressure applied to the specific areas on the hands or feet increases or decreases energy in another area of the body. Most often reflexology is performed on the feet although some practitioners will also work on the hands or even the ears. The concepts of reflexology can be traced to Egypt, Japan, China, and elsewhere in the East where massage of the feet was associated with therapeutic benefit for the whole person. Modern day reflexology arose from a twentieth-century practice called Zone Therapy. Drawing on the Eastern theories, William Fitzgerald, an American physician, is reported to have observed anesthetic benefits associated with pressure points on the feet. He created a ten-zone map of the feet that related to other areas of the body. Eunice Ingham, a physical therapist and nurse, expanded on Fitzgerald's theory and is credited with producing the reflexology map of the feet. This map of the soles, sides, and top of the feet created a mirror of the body. Other practitioners created energy-zone maps of the hands and ears but this is a less common practice.

A typical reflexology treatment is applied to the feet. It is performed with the client fully clothed except for bare feet. The client sits in a reclined or recumbent position. Depending on the practitioner, a pre-session interview and health history survey may be used, but it is not required. The treatment usually begins with kneading, shaking, and stretching the foot, ankle, and toes to relax the feet. Then a systematic sequence of thumb and finger pressure is applied to the feet. One hand is used to support the foot while pressure is applied with the other hand. The special technique associated with reflexology involves pressure and movement of the thumbs or fingers known as crawling or walking. The movement is pressing, bending, and releasing the thumb as it moves over the foot. It resembles an inchworm and is performed in specific patterns over the individual zones. Direct sustained pressure, stroking, and kneading are sometimes used, but the basic technique involves crawling or walking with the thumbs. The practitioner may alternate working on the feet or work on one foot entirely before moving to the other.

The goal of the treatment is to release energy blockages in areas associated with organs of the body that are not functioning properly. Assessment is often part of the treatment. Although clients are usually relaxed during the treatment, sometimes a dialogue with the practitioner is helpful to uncover why a specific area of the foot feels different. Often the areas of the feet that correspond with the client's health issues will be tender, sore, or tight compared to other areas of the foot.

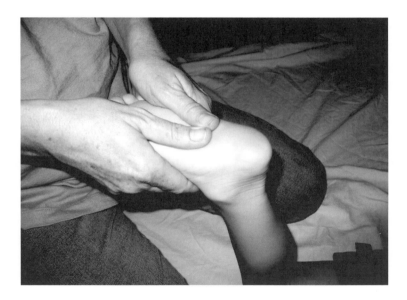

Figure 8.1 Reflexology

The treatment sequence can be general reflexology for relaxation or created to address specific organs of the body that relate to a health problem. General reflexology would include pressure to the major organ systems such as the brain, digestive, circulatory, and respiratory systems. For example, a client with asthma would receive pressure to the areas of the foot that correspond with the heart and lungs. Pressure may also be applied to general zones of the feet to encourage relaxation (see Figure 8.1). A typical reflexology session lasts about one hour, but can range from ten to ninety minutes. Techniques may be added to a conventional massage session or spa treatment, such as a facial. Because reflexology works on one region of the body, it is well suited to short treatments.

Research on reflexology has produced some interesting results. Several studies have found that it is associated with increased relaxation and reduced anxiety. However, reflexology has not produced significantly more benefit when compared to general foot massage. There is little research to substantiate the benefits of reflexology or pressure to specific energy zones on the function of the target organs. The overall conclusions from the body of research suggest that massaging or performing reflexology on the feet can have a positive impact on the whole person.

For individuals with ASD, the amount of sensory information from the feet or hands may be too much to process or understand. As pointed out earlier in the book, this is illustrated by behaviors like toe-walking so that the feet do not fully touch the ground or touching objects with the back of the hand rather than the palm and fingers. Reflexology may be very useful for clients with this type of sensory problem. The systematic application of touch can help to improve touch receptivity through use of a predictable pattern of touch and careful modification of pressure. Treatment of the zones associated with the brain, spinal column, nervous system, and endocrine glands may also produce a calming effect. Reflexology or even just hand or foot massage may also benefit sensory issues because the touch is applied to a localized area of the body. Beginning a touch therapy with a small area may train a client to learn to feel and process touch.

This could serve as a gateway to improve touch receptivity to a larger area of the body over time.

POLARITY THERAPY

Polarity Therapy is a holistic approach toward healing. It blends knowledge of Western science with energetic bodywork, nutritional recommendations, lifestyle counseling and corrective exercises to promote the balance and flow of energy. Polarity Therapy was developed in the 1950s by Randolph Stone, an osteopathic physician. Dr. Stone traveled extensively and studied different healing techniques around the world. He recognized the presence of negative and positive energy in the body as well as areas that were perceived as neutral.

Stone drew from similarities found in many of the forms of healing he studied. His work combined theories used in ayurveda in India with Traditional Chinese Medicine to understand and treat illness and disease. In ayurveda there are seven different energy centers in the body (*chakras*). Energy of a person and the environment are found in different forces of the *air, water, earth, fire,* and *ether.* There are three different types of energy: quick (*rajas*), heavy (*tamas*), and still (*sattva*). In Traditional Chinese Medicine there are five elements of energy (*fire, earth, metal, water,* and *wood*) and fourteen energy pathways that correspond with organs of the body. *Yin* and *yang* represent the different flows of opposing forces of energy. Stone also found similarities between these expressions of energy and the traditional sign representing the Western or allopathic physician. His goal was to integrate different theories into a comprehensive healing modality.

Polarity Therapy explores the balance of energy on different dimensions. Before treatment, the practitioner will conduct an interview with the client and a holistic evaluation.

This includes observing the client's appearance, mannerisms, voice, and posture. The practitioner will also check qualities of the client's pulse on the neck and ankles. The five elements of energy in Polarity Therapy (air, water, earth, fire, or ether) represent different qualities of energy. The energy in the center of the body is believed to be neutral; energy on other areas of the body flows between positive and negative poles. Polarity Therapy also recognizes the roles of internal organs and cerebrospinal fluid in promoting and restoring health. When energy is blocked it affects the physiological function of the body. The goal of an evaluation is to identify which energy element is blocked and work with the client to restore energy flow.

A Polarity Therapy session can last 60–90 minutes. Because there are many different approaches used in Polarity Therapy, the components of the session are different. For a hands-on Polarity Therapy treatment, the client is positioned on a massage table either fully or partially clothed and covered with a sheet or blanket. Different areas of the body are related to the five different energy elements. The practitioner places his or her hands on areas related to a specific element. The hands are positioned at two different locations on the client's body to feel the energy that flows between the hands. Different touch techniques including kneading, rubbing, rocking, or stroking may be used to stimulate energy flow. The pace of the session is dependent on the practitioner's sense of the client's energy current. Polarity Therapy practitioners are trained to sense the pulses and quality of energy. During a session the practitioner works with a specific area until he or she feels a change in energy flow and then moves on to another area.

There is little research on Polarity Therapy to date. Polarity Therapy treatments depend on the practitioner's evaluation of the client. That may be different depending on the practitioner. The inclusion of counseling, nutritional recommendations and exercises in Polarity Therapy as well as bodywork and touch suggests that the benefits may be achieved from this holistic approach.

Since Polarity Therapy includes touch techniques as well as energy work, it may be beneficial for individuals with ASD on a few levels. The stimulation from the touch may help meet sensory needs and encourage positive reception to touch. The possibility for energy work to aid in healing an imbalance is an important potential for any energy therapy. Another aspect of Polarity Therapy is the holistic approach that includes corrective exercises and nutritional counseling. The practitioner may be able to work with a client with ASD and their caregiver to identify exercises or stretches that could meet stimulation needs in a positive way. It is also possible that the nutritional problems often found with ASD could be viewed from an energy-related perspective. If so, then a Polarity Therapy practitioner may help to identify foods that could help meet nutritional and energy flow needs.

Traditional energy-based massage

In traditional settings, holistic medicine practitioners treat patients using a variety of techniques. These may include: massage, herbal medicines, acupuncture, moxibustion (burning an herb called mugwort), herbal compresses, nutritional therapy, spiritual counseling, and exercise prescription. In areas of the world where traditional medicine is considered CAM, laws and regulations can affect the practice of traditional medicine. Often this limits CAM practitioners in their legal scope of practice. This means that a licensed or certified massage practitioner may not legally offer nutritional counseling, perform acupuncture, or prescribe herbal remedies.

Tuina

A traditional massage from China called tuina is based on an ancient massage form called *anma*. References to the therapeutic use of massage date far back in history. One reference is the *Neijing*, a classic text on Traditional Chinese Medicine. Anma, the massage approach at that time, was the predecessor to Tuina. Anma is reported to have included massage techniques using the hands and special tools, along with herbs and prescribed exercise to treat various illnesses. Acupuncture, herbal medicine, and massage are the three components of Traditional Chinese Medicine. Around the time of the Ming Dynasty in the mid-fourteenth century, anma gave rise to tuina, which appeared as a specialized aspect of traditional medicine.

The practice of tuina existed for centuries; instruction on tuina was passed on through the generations by mentoring. Massage was applied to treat a wide range of medical conditions including muscle pain, gynecological problems, and digestive disorders such as constipation and diarrhea. The principles used in tuina are taken from Traditional Chinese Medicine. Illness and disease are viewed as imbalances of energy. The name tuina translates to mean *lift-press*. An abundance of strokes and manipulation techniques are used to reduce or reinforce the flow of chi in the body depending on the condition being treated. Tuina is considered to be a forerunner of European medical gymnastics that would eventually give rise to Swedish massage. The creation of tuina training programs in China in the mid-twentieth century helped to legitimize tuina as a form of healthcare.

Massage and Traditional Chinese Medicine as well as medicine throughout Asia were concerned with the flow of energy. Concepts of Traditional Chinese Medicine center on the five elements of nature (*fire, earth, metal, water,* and *wood*) and the balance of energy (*chi*). Chi is expressed as a continuum that flows to create perpetual balance. People are born with chi, but also can get it from food and air which are necessary to sustain life. Good health requires an adequate amount of balanced chi throughout the lifetime. When chi is depleted or out of balance (too much in one area, too little in another) it can lead to illness or disease. A person's spirit (*shen*) and their essence (*jing*) contribute to their character and to their health.

There are fourteen energy pathways (*meridians*) and 365 energy points (*tsubos*) that are associated with specific organs of the body. The meridians are paired to form a balance of *yin* and *yang* energy and are arranged within one of the five elements of nature. Yin and yang represent a balance of opposite types of energy found in the universe. They can be understood as expressing concepts like dark/light, masculine/feminine, or passive/active. Different physical and psychological characteristics are associated with normal manifestations of chi as well as energy imbalances.

An easy meridian to understand and trace is the Heart meridian. Trace a path from the center of the armpit along the front of the arm, past the inside of the elbow, across the side of the palm of the hand, to the end of the small finger. This is the heart meridian. Specific points on the meridian include Heart 1 (in the center of the armpit), Heart 3 (on the corner of the crease in the elbow), Heart 7 (on the corner of the wrist crease), and Heart 9 (near the bottom of the nail on the small finger).

Tuina sessions usually last an hour. The client is positioned on a massage table or raised futon and may be fully or partially clothed. Massage techniques used in tuina include kneading, rubbing, stroking, twisting, vibration, percussion, stretching, and joint mobilization. Use of the hands, fists, fingers, forearms, and elbows creates many options to adjust the amount of pressure applied to a particular area. The massage is applied to specific areas of the body including the head, ears, abdomen, as well as the back, arms, and legs. The areas of the body are selected because of the location of meridians that lack or have too much chi.

Traditional Chinese Medicine meridians travel across different areas of the body. Therefore there is an opportunity for a *referred* benefit. For example, many children with ASD have feeding and eating-related problems. In these cases the stomach meridian is important. It flows from the eye down the front of the body, across the abdomen, and down the leg to the second toe. If children will not tolerate touch to their face, feet, or abdomen, massage and stretching applied to the leg can help the flow of stomach-related chi.

Drawing conclusions about the benefits of tuina for ASD is difficult, because tuina is often used along with other traditional therapies including cupping and moxibustion. This is apparent in many of the research studies that have attempted to evaluate the benefits of tuina. Understanding ASD in the context of Traditional Chinese Medicine is complex because it likely involves subtle imbalances of chi in several different elements and meridians.[23] Because traditional medicine takes a complex and holistic view of health, treatment recommendations can vary tremendously. This includes the design of a single massage session.

There are many different techniques used in tuina that offer sensory benefit for an individual with ASD. Stretches and joint mobilization may help with proprioceptive awareness and tight muscles. As with any massage style, massage strokes and pressure can increase touch receptivity. There are a wide variety of techniques and stretches used in tuina, which offers many possibilities for a child with ASD. This rather diverse approach to hands-on therapy gives the practitioner many tools to work with in experimenting on tuina as a sensory intervention.

Shiatsu

Shiatsu is a form of bodywork from Japan that uses pressure to promote the flow of chi. Translated as "finger pressure," the theory that forms the foundation for shiatsu is based on principles used in acupuncture and tuina. The origins of shiatsu can be traced to Traditional Chinese Medicine and anma which was a form of massage performed by blind practitioners in Japan. The practice of shiatsu evolved in Japan to integrate aspects of Western anatomy and physiology with traditional teachings of health.

The beginnings of Shiatsu practice in Western countries happened in the mid-twentieth century. There are different schools of thought in shiatsu concerned with the evaluation of the flow of chi and the approach to shiatsu massage treatment. Two of the basic forms are derived from Nippon-style and Zen shiatsu. Nippon-style shiatsu was developed by Tokujiro Namikoshi, who founded a massage school in Japan after World War II. He integrated Western anatomy and physiology into sessions that used systematic thumb and palm pressure along energy pathways (*meridians*) and on points (*tsubos*). Zen shiatsu was developed by one of Namikoshi's students, Shizuto Masunaga. He developed a practice in the 1970s that focused on the spiritual aspects of energy and de-emphasized Western scientific explanations for health and disease. Masunaga focused on meridians rather than points and also expanded the traditional meridians to include extensions over more areas on the body. Namikoshi and Masunaga's approaches to shiatsu have given rise to many different interpretations and forms of shiatsu practice. A common theme among all interpretations of shiatsu is the concern with the flow of chi. Chi flows along fourteen energy meridians and through 365 points. Shiatsu aims to create a balance by dispersing the excessive energy and nurturing in the deficient area.

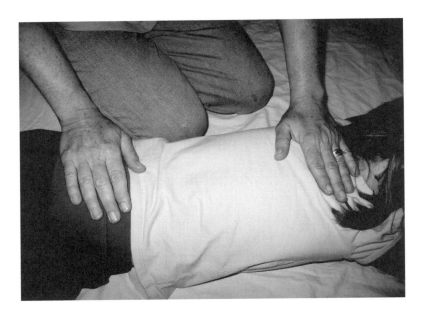

Figure 8.2 Shiatsu

The client is fully clothed for a shiatsu session, which can be performed on a futon, floor mat, or massage table (see Figure 8.2). Shiatsu practitioners take different approaches to massage treatment. A holistic pre-massage assessment may be performed. This may include a health history, lifestyle questionnaire, visual observation, and touch assessment. Touch can be used to evaluate energy on any of the meridians, but evaluation of the abdomen is important. The abdomen is considered to be the center of a person's energy. The energy zones on the abdomen (called the *hara*) correspond to the twelve energetic meridians. Pressing the area enables the practitioner to feel the core of the client's energy. The goal of the evaluation is to assess energy on multiple levels including how it looks, feels, sounds, and even smells. Regardless of the methods used to evaluate the client's energy, the goal of shiatsu is to facilitate the flow of energy along the meridians.

So the energy evaluation often continues during the massage as the practitioner senses shifts in energy in response to the massage.

Shiatsu is a flexible form of bodywork. The shiatsu practitioner may apply a general massage to promote energy balance or design a specific treatment that he or she believes will best meet the needs of the client. The selection of meridians, points, and style of pressure can be tailored to promote energy flow in specific areas of the body. Two-handed contact is used while the practitioner performs palm, finger, or thumb pressure along the meridians. Elbow, knee, or foot pressure, stretches, joint mobilization, and percussive techniques may also be used. The quality of pressure can be adapted to be slow, vigorous, light, or deep. Although the meridians flow along the surface of the body, a person's energy is also deep. Shiatsu pressure penetrates deep into the body. It is important for the practitioner to remain relaxed to maintain focus on and connection with the client. A typical shiatsu treatment lasts about one hour, but shorter or longer sessions can be performed.

Research has found that shiatsu can help with pain relief, promote relaxation and feelings of overall well-being. However, there are inconsistencies in shiatsu research regarding the techniques used as well as the length and frequency of treatment sessions. To date shiatsu has not been evaluated for ASD. It may be beneficial in a number of ways. Shiatsu uses a variety of types of pressure, stretching, and joint movements. This can offer additional techniques beyond those typically incorporated in sensory therapy sessions. It may help meet sensory needs and improve receptivity to touch. Shiatsu can also address imbalances of the flow of chi which may help modulate the nervous system and help individuals with ASD feel relaxed.

Qi gong massage

Qi gong is a system of breathing and movement from China that aims to increase the flow of energy. There are many different interpretations of qi gong (also called chi kung or chi gung). It can be practiced as a form of meditation, for physical training, or to promote or restore health. Most often qi gong is practiced as meditative exercise, in a manner similar to martial arts. This method traditionally involves active movement, holding static postures or poses, visualization or meditation techniques, or self-massage. Stretching, pressure, and massage techniques, similar to tuina and shiatsu, can also be practiced using qi gong principles.

Qi gong massage is also referred to as meridian therapy or acupressure. The theories of the meridians of Traditional Chinese Medicine that are used in tuina and shiatsu provide the foundation for qi gong massage. The pathways (meridians) and points (tsubos) on the body contain the energy of life (qi or chi). When a person is physically, psychologically, and emotionally healthy energy flows in an unobstructed manner. Disease or illness is associated with disturbances in the flow of chi. It may be blocked, stagnant, or lacking on meridians or points that are associated with different organs of the body. Various stretching, exercise, or massage techniques can be used to release energy blockages and promote energy flow.

The theory and application of qi gong massage is very similar to tuina and shiatsu. A qi gong massage is performed with the client fully clothed, lying on a futon, mat, or massage table. The length of a qi gong massage session can vary from just a few minutes to one hour. An energy evaluation and health interview is performed prior to the massage. Based on information from the client and the practitioner's observation, a massage treatment is designed to treat specific energy pathways and points. A difference in qi gong massage is that it may include energy work that involves very light touch with the hands or fingers. This touch aims to gently manipulate the flow of qi on a very subtle level. The practitioner may ask the client to engage in deep breathing exercises to encourage emotional release of blocked energy.

A series of research studies on qi gong massage for individuals with ASD noted improvements in sensory measurements, sleep, and social skills.[24–27] Over time, the children became more receptive to touch. These findings suggest benefits for qi gong massage and general benefits for massage as a complementary therapy. Because there are similarities in the theory and techniques, a difficulty with qi gong massage involves differentiating this style from tuina, acupressure, and shiatsu. The positive research findings suggest that there can be benefit for massage styles that are based on similar methods. Like research on Swedish massage for ASD, the qi gong massage research protocols involved teaching parents to massage their children. Performing a short massage daily made the massage part of the child's regular sensory therapy. This offers parents and caregivers an extra tool in helping to meet sensory needs.

Thai massage

Thai massage is a traditional form of massage from Thailand. It is part of the indigenous medical system along with nutrition, herbs, and spiritual healing. The basis for traditional Thai medicine is attributed to Buddha's personal physician, Jivaka. The modern origins of Thai medicine can be traced to the mid-thirteenth century. It is a holistic approach to healthcare that draws components from medical practices from China and India as well as Buddhism. Theravada Buddhism is the most popular religion of Thailand. Compassion and kindness are central to its teachings. The practice of Thai medicine is in line with concepts from Theravada Buddhism. It aimed to promote health of Thai people in a compassionate way that was respectful to ancestors and nature.[28]

Thailand encourages religious freedom but Buddhism has had a longstanding influence on Thai culture. There are over 25,000 temples (*wats*) scattered throughout Thailand. For centuries Thai Buddhist monasteries and temples were centers for education and healing. This included spiritual practices and the arts of traditional medicine. Information about Thai traditional medicine was passed down orally and in written form. In the early nineteenth century, information about Thai medicine and massage was carved into stone and statues at two temples (Wat Pho and Wat Raja Oros) in Bangkok. Medical texts are said to have been as important and revered as spiritual texts.

According to Thai medical beliefs, the body is made up of four elements (*tards*): earth, wind, fire, and water. Optimal health requires a balance of these elements. Illness or disease is associated with an imbalance of energy that can be caused by the universe, pathogens, forces of nature, or supernatural power. Herbal remedies, spiritual healing, and massage were prescribed to restore the balance of energy. Thai medicine began to be practiced outside of the temples. Over time, Thai medicine evolved so that its teachings and traditions were interpreted in different ways.

The introduction of Western (allopathic) medicine to Thailand in the mid-nineteenth century brought understanding of anatomy and physiology which added a new dimension to Thai medicine. The first Western-style medical school that was opened in Bangkok initially taught traditional and Western medicine, but ultimately stopped teaching Thai medicine. This led to changes in healthcare laws which made it illegal for many traditional practitioners to work. Traditional Thai medicine was still practiced in rural areas and a growing interest developed in the 1970s.

Medical schools were opened in Thailand to teach traditional medicine. A government economic stimulus helped to fund the opening of massage schools to train massage practitioners. Interest from Western tourists in yoga and massage led to the development of massage schools around Thailand.

Thai massage integrates concepts from traditional medicine with anatomy and physiology. It is not a religious practice, but its rocking movements, pressure, and stretching techniques are performed in a rhythmic manner which can be meditative. In this way it is said to benefit the practitioner as well as the client. Thai massage is performed on a floor mat or low futon with the client fully clothed, except for bare feet. Sessions can last between one and two hours. In a full session the client is positioned in different ways including lying prone (on the stomach), supine (on the back), side-lying and seated. The changes in position give the practitioner the ability to easily touch and stretch different areas of the body (see Figure 8.3 for neck massage). Fundamental to Thai massage are the ten energy pathways (*sen*) on the body. Massage techniques aim to promote the flow of energy along the sen lines. There are two basic styles of Thai massage. Northern-style (also known as folk massage) uses pressure applied by the hands, fists, knees, or feet along with stretches. Royal massage uses finger and hand pressure on points on the sen lines. Oil is not used for Thai massage, but herbal compresses are sometimes used.

Traditionally massage was used to treat a variety of disorders. Regular massage aims to promote the flow of energy throughout the body and can be used in rehabilitation of illnesses or injuries. Massage protocols for specific health problems pay significant attention to the abdomen. Many of the sen lines are found on the abdomen and it is also considered to be the place that is the origin of the body's air. The wide variety of stretches in Thai massage encourages flexibility of joints in multiple directions.

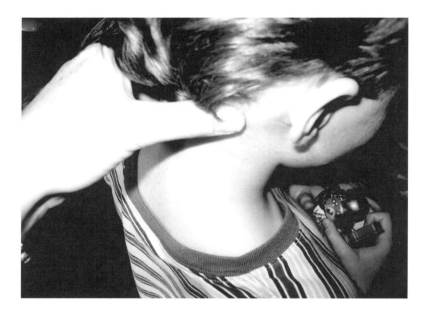

Figure 8.3 Thai massage

Research suggests that Thai massage can be beneficial for individuals with ASD.[29] The variety of techniques and repertoire of stretches offer potential benefits for proprioceptive needs and could also help areas of muscle tightness or imbalances. Some of the techniques combine pressure and stretching in a way that is distinctly similar to myofascial release. Although the theory behind the technique is different in these styles, the potential benefit is the same. Because Thai massage is performed with the client clothed and on the floor, it puts a child with ASD in a comfortable and safe position to receive touch.

ACUPRESSURE-BASED BODYWORK

Acupressure is a term that is used in different ways to describe various approaches to massage and bodywork. Sometimes it is used as a general term that includes Eastern forms of massage such as shiatsu and tuina. There are many forms of massage and bodywork that incorporate acupressure techniques or theories of Traditional Chinese Medicine. Some are purported to be rediscovered ancient therapies. Other styles combine acupressure with concepts from Western anatomy and physiology. Some interpretation of the concept of chi is usually associated with acupressure.

Jin Shin Jyutsu®

Jin Shin Jyutsu® is a style of bodywork based on ancient massage that is reported to have been rediscovered by Jiro Murai in Japan in the early twentieth century. Various forms of massage in Japan integrated concepts of Traditional Chinese Medicine along with Taoist and Buddhist explanations for health and illness with Japanese massage techniques. Murai believed that the flow of chi was important for health. He developed a system that used pressure on acupuncture points and channels along with exercises and stretches. His use of specific hand positions and sequences aimed to promote the flow of chi and of body fluids. Murai referred to his work as an art that brought balance and harmony. He taught his methods in an informal way in Japan. One of his students, Mary Lino Burmeister, moved to the United States and created Jin Shin Jyutsu® based on his teachings.

A Jin Shin Jyutsu® session is one hour. It is performed with the client clothed, lying face up on a futon or massage table. To begin the massage the practitioner evaluates the client's pulse at the wrist. Then the practitioner designs a series of hand positions (*flows*) applied to specific points on the body. Very light touch is used to promote the flow of chi. The aim of the session is to use various combinations of hand positions to unlock tension.

ASD is not known to be associated with specific patterns of the flow of chi. This is illustrated by the many different presentations across the ASD spectrum. Massage styles that use light touch may increase touch receptivity and have a calming effect for some individuals, but may be irritating to others. For an individual with ASD who is very sensitive to touch, Jin Shin Jyutsu® may provide a systematic way to balance chi and provide a soothing sensory stimulus.

Jin Shin Do®

Jin Shin Do® is a form of massage that integrates theories and techniques from Jin Shin Jyutsu® as well as several other styles of bodywork. It was developed in California in the 1970s by a psychotherapist, Iona Teeguarden. She studied Jin Shin Jyutsu® with Mary Burmeister and studied various approaches to acupressure. Teeguarden was a marriage and family therapist who explored psychotherapeutic benefits of bodywork. She created her own style of bodywork that incorporated theory and techniques of Jin Shin Jyutsu.® Teeguarden also incorporated the philosophy of Milton Erickson (known for specializing in hypnosis) and Wilhelm Reich (who wrote about repressed emotions and psychosexual energy) into her work.

Jin Shin Do® is performed with the client lying face up on a massage table. Sessions can last either sixty or ninety minutes. Jin Shin Do® uses fifty-five points from acupuncture called acu-points. These points are located in common areas of muscle tension and are also integral to the flow of chi. The practitioner assesses the client's tension patterns by evaluating the pulse and by sensing acu-points. A Jin Shin Do® session aims to release areas of habitual tension (armoring) through massage techniques and exercises along with verbal counseling. The points are pressed or held in various combinations for several minutes. Jin Shin Do® uses hard and soft pressure depending on the point and the type of tension. Clients are encouraged to talk about how a point feels to help them understand the meaning behind tension and to encourage psychological and physical release of tension.

The importance of the client being aware of and understanding muscle tension is integral to Jin Shin Do.® An individual with ASD would not likely have a sophisticated awareness. However, the integral relationship between the mind and the body that is central to Jin Shin Do® suggests that it may benefit a person with ASD on a psychological and a sensory level.

Amma therapy

Amma therapy is a bodywork style that integrates Eastern and Western techniques for health and disease with pressure and stroking massage techniques. It was developed in the 1970s by Tina Sohn. She learned about Korean folk medicine and acupuncture from her grandmother, who helped her to heal after an accident. Ms. Sohn was also an intuitive who could sense people's pains and illnesses. She studied healing in Korea and moved to the United States in the mid-1960s. Her husband, an American acupuncturist, herbalist, and martial arts enthusiast, opened a holistic health school. Ms. Sohn began teaching the bodywork style that grew out of her studies.

Amma therapy integrates concepts of Traditional Chinese Medicine with knowledge of anatomy and physiology from Western medicine, and concepts of reflexology. Pre-massage assessment is an important component in Amma therapy. The practitioner interviews the client about lifestyle, habits, and health problems. The practitioner will also observe the client and touch (palpate) different areas of the body to sense energy. The aim of the assessment is to create a portrait of the client's mind and body and understand the energy imbalance that is unique to each client.

During an Amma therapy session, the client lies on a massage table wearing loose comfortable clothing. The length of the session can vary, but is usually one hour. Different types of techniques are used in Amma therapy to balance chi along the channels or energy pathways (meridians). Massage techniques draw from Swedish massage, Shiatsu, reflexology, and Structural Integration. Stroking, deep and soft pressure, joint manipulations, stretching, and kneading may be incorporated into the session.

Like other energy-based therapies, Amma therapy may offer potential benefit to individuals with ASD. It has not been evaluated as a therapeutic intervention to date. The holistic assessment makes it possible to consider the different sensory and psychological issues in the context of an imbalance of chi. Amma practitioners use a broad array of techniques that are drawn from other modalities. In that way, Amma therapy is somewhat eclectic. The technique menu offers the practitioner many different choices and approaches to touch.

NON-CONTACT ENERGY THERAPIES

Non-contact energy therapies are types of bodywork that do not use manipulation of muscles. They may not even actually involve touch. They attempt to manipulate the human energy field by placing the hands close to or lightly on the body. A license or certification is not required for most non-contact therapies, so they are widely used by healthcare and wellness practitioners who are not eligible for a massage license or certification. Although there is much enthusiasm for non-contact therapies, research on the benefits of these therapies has been mixed.[30–33]

Therapeutic Touch

Therapeutic Touch is a form of energy healing that involves no actual contact. The practitioner places his or her hands on or close to the client to project energy toward the client. The intention behind the healing is viewed as important. The underlying assumptions behind Therapeutic Touch include the beliefs that there is a human energy field, energy imbalances are related to illness or disease, and the energy can be felt and stimulated. The stimulation of energy involves releasing and moving blocked energy. This is accomplished through the placement and direction of the practitioner's hands.

A popular therapy with nurses, Therapeutic Touch was developed in the 1970s by Dolores Krieger, a nurse, and Dora Kunz, a spiritual and natural healer. They aimed to promote nurse-patient relationships by using a non-religious laying on of the hands. Early Therapeutic Touch sessions involved actually touching the recipient, but the practice evolved to a non-contact approach. Short sessions could be incorporated into regular nursing duties and brought a holistic aspect to nursing care. Some of the theory behind Therapeutic Touch is taken from ayurveda, including the description of energy as *prana* and energy centers as *chakras*.

Therapeutic Touch sessions have a series of steps. Clients are fully clothed and can be in any position to receive a session, depending on their state of health. Traditionally, the client is in a seated position on a stool, bench, or sideways in a chair so that the back can be accessed. The practitioner begins by *centering* to clear his or her mind of distractions and focus on the patient. Depending on the practitioner, the centering process may involve a short meditation or breathing practice. The goal is to turn the attention inward, adopt a relaxed presence, and create an open mind. This aids the practitioner in focusing on the present moment and the goal of healing. The practitioner creates an intention of healing. The healing intention is believed to be an important aspect of Therapeutic Touch treatment.

Centering is followed by an *energetic assessment* from the client's head to feet. Energy is believed to flow from the head downwards, so the session begins with the practitioner's hands over the top of the client's head. The hands are typically held two to four inches away from the client's body. The practitioner moves his or her hands down the client's body toward the feet feeling for changes in energy. These changes are referred to as cues that there is an energy blockage. Healthy energy is perceived as smooth and symmetrical. Cues that there are energy imbalances include pulsing, tingling, pulling or pushing sensations, changes in temperature, or even an intuition. The energy assessment can be performed first on the back of the body then the front, or simultaneously on the front and back of the body with the practitioner standing by the client's side.

The assessment is followed by a clearing process called *unruffling*. The practitioner uses brushing motions to remove energy clusters or disturbances by sweeping the energy towards the client's feet. Once the energy is perceived as cleared, the practitioner directs energy to areas where imbalances were felt during the assessment. The practitioner's hands are placed on opposite sides of the body so that energy can be directed between the hands using rebalancing or modulation techniques. For *rebalancing*, the practitioner directs an opposite energy toward the area of disturbance. For example, firm energy would be directed toward an area that is soft or weak. *Modulation* manipulates the client's own energy by smoothing it out. The practitioner may visualize colors to project toward the client.

Sessions can be relatively short, even a few minutes. A session ends when the practitioner feels that the client's energy is in better balance. Assessment of the client's energy occurs throughout the session and relies heavily on the practitioner's intuitive sense and focus on the client.

Research on Therapeutic Touch is somewhat inconclusive. It is associated with decreased anxiety and increased feelings of relaxation and well-being. However, studies have not been able to substantiate the practitioner's ability to "feel" energy or the benefits of Therapeutic Touch compared to a "sham" treatment that lacked healing intention. The non-contact aspect of Therapeutic Touch does not directly treat any sensory needs for an individual with ASD. However, it is not likely to cause any harm.

Healing Touch

Healing Touch is a non-contact energy-based therapy that has its roots in nursing practice. It was developed in the 1980s by a nurse, Janet Mentgen, as a nurturing therapy offered as continuing education for nurses. Healing Touch is based on concepts from other healers and scientists and is recognized by the American Holistic Nursing Association for continuing education. The theories of Healing Touch draw on the chakras from ayurveda and include references to modern medicine. It is described as a heart-centered and caring approach to healthcare practice. Intention is essential for a Healing Touch session and the relationship between the practitioner and client is an important aspect of treatment. The goal is to work with the client's own energy to promote physical, mental, and emotional balance. The practitioner works as a facilitator in order to help the client heal him or herself. It takes a whole-person view of bodywork rather than focus on one area of illness or disease.

A Healing Touch session can last up to one hour. It begins with a pre-treatment *consultation*. The practitioner interviews the client about his or her physical, mental, and emotional health. The client is fully clothed for a Healing Touch treatment and lies on a massage table. The practitioner centers him or herself prior to the treatment. This may be done by a variety of ways including breathing exercises, meditation, or even prayer. Centering helps the practitioner to ignore distractions and focus on the client. The practitioner uses his or her hands to scan and manipulate the client's energy. The hands are positioned a few inches away from the client or may lightly touch the client.

The practitioner's hands are used to evaluate the client's energy, restore symmetry to the energy, and open the client's chakras. Different techniques are used to feel and manipulate energy including magnetic passes, pain draining, wound sealing, mind clearing, energetic ultrasound and energy lasers. Excess energy is directed downward and outward away from the client. Throughout the session, the practitioner continues to evaluate changes in the client's energy.

Although the body of evidence is inconclusive, research suggests that clients can benefit from receiving Healing Touch. Research has noted that clients feel relaxed and less anxious after a session. Healing Touch does not provide any sensory stimulation that would benefit an individual with ASD. Since it is a non-invasive body therapy, there is little risk to the client.

Reiki

Reiki is a form of energy healing that uses laying on of hands, sounds, symbols, and mantras in treatment. It also has a series of life principles called *ideals*. Although the origins of Reiki are from Japan and the East, it is not considered to be a traditional form of bodywork. Rather it was developed in the late 1800s based on interpretations of Eastern theories of health and healing. Reiki addresses the flow of energy known as *chi* (also spelled *qi* or *ki*). When there is a lack of energy or poor flow, it causes illness or disease. Peace and harmony are fundamental to Reiki.

Reiki is not connected to a religion, but its origins are reported to have arisen out of exploration of miracle healing. The practice of Reiki was developed by Mikao Usui, a Christian minister teaching in Japan. Interested in the use of hands-on healing in Christianity, Usui explored similar concepts in Buddhism. He began to use hands-on healing techniques after he had a mystical experience during meditation. Over the years Usui's techniques evolved as they were interpreted by his students. Hawayo Takata received Reiki from one of Usui's student successors. She is credited for bringing Reiki to the West in the early twentieth century and training many Reiki masters.

Reiki practitioners work to increase a client's chi and the flow of chi by using their own energy as a conduit. Although many Eastern traditions view chi as universal life energy, for Reiki practitioners the chi must be unlocked by a Reiki master through a process called *attunement*. This process takes several stages of treatment (*degree*) by a Reiki master. A treatment delivered by a Reiki practitioner will depend on his or her degree of attunement. The principles or ideals of Reiki require that the practitioner be healthy and connected to his or her own chi. A new Reiki practitioner is trained to perform Reiki using approximately a dozen specific hand positions over the chakras and organs of the body. Advanced practitioners can practice distance healing with Reiki through the use of symbols and images to form a bridge between the practitioner and the client. Humming sounds and repeated healing words (*mantras*) are sometimes used to aid in healing.

Reiki sessions are performed on fully clothed clients. The client can be positioned in any manner that is comfortable. Session lengths vary and can last up to ninety minutes. Energetic assessment is not necessary for a Reiki session. The practitioner begins by placing his or her hands at the top of the head and the treatment progresses down toward the feet. As different areas of the body are treated, the client is expected to experience tingling and other sensations including changes in temperature. The Reiki practitioner intuitively treats different areas of the body based on the feel of the client's chi.

As a non-invasive treatment, Reiki is not dangerous. It does not require touch, but the client may feel sensations. Therefore, it could benefit individuals with ASD. Research suggests that Reiki may be beneficial for pain and stress reduction and to promote relaxation. However, studies have not successfully provided evidence to substantiate many of the suggested outcomes or the overall benefit of Reiki.

9
Other Styles of Touch-Based Therapeutic Bodywork

Although massage is thought of as passive, some forms of bodywork involve the participation of the client. Educating the client about movement, alignment, and reactions to stress are often important. The styles and modalities that fall within the category of therapeutic bodywork can be extremely broadened or narrowed as needed. Movement-based modalities and activities that are self-initiated are not included here. Since the focus of this book is on touch and sensation, styles that include some form of touch are described. The styles that are discussed in this chapter are some of the more established or unique modalities that offer potential benefit for individuals with ASDs.

WATSU®

Watsu® is pool-based treatment that integrates principles of shiatsu and aquatic therapy. Stretches and pressure are performed with the client floating in a shallow, heated pool. The client's body is supported by the practitioner and buoyed by the water and sometimes flotation devices. The warmth of the water and the supported position of the body combine to relax the mind and body to alleviate muscle tension. Watsu® was created in the early 1980s by Harold Dull, a Shiatsu teacher. Dull floated his shiatsu students in water. He applied shiatsu stretches and pressure and noticed that the body could stretch in a wider variety of positions in water than it could on dry land. As with other forms of aquatic therapy, immersion in water reduced stress on joints while providing resistance in movement. The pressure of the water increases awareness of the body and the position of the joints. As Dull's technique developed over time, he added breathing exercises to encourage relaxation and self-awareness.

A Watsu® session lasts 45–60 minutes. Prior to the session, the practitioner interviews the client about health and medical conditions. Muscle and joint range-of-motion tests may be conducted prior to entering the water. The client and practitioner wear bathing suits. After entering the water, flotation devices may be placed around the ankles or under the body. The practitioner moves, rocks, and stretches the client while supporting the client's head above the water. At the end of the session, the client is assisted in standing upright.

A survey on the possible benefits of aquatic therapy for children with Autism suggested that muscle strength, balance, and touch receptiveness improved after aquatic therapy.[34] Although aquatic therapy is recommended for children with developmental disabilities or neuromuscular disorders, there is little research evidence that it improves strength, coordination, or flexibility.[35,36] Unlike aquatic therapy, Watsu® is passive movement in water. Therefore it is not likely to improve muscle tone or strength as would be expected with aquatic therapy that involves actual exercise in water. Immersion in water does stimulate the tactile sense and moving in water provides stimulation of the joints. The warmth and support of the water during a Watsu® session does offer possibilities of increased range of motion in stretches. An individual with ASD who does enjoy being in the water may be more receptive to touch in a warm pool. Being held, rocked, and stretched may be comforting for some clients.

FELDENKRAIS®

The Feldenkrais Method® is a movement-based form of bodywork that aims to train the body to move efficiently. There are two basic aspects of Feldenkrais.® One involves active movements, the other is touch and passive movement performed by the practitioner. The active movement approach to Feldenkrais® is called Awareness Through Movement.® The practitioner uses verbal cues to instruct the client in performing movements. The passive approach in Feldenkrais® is called Functional Integration.® This involves a range of motion movements and stretches that are performed by the practitioner. The goal of Feldenkrais® is to educate people on how they can move, stand, and sit properly without any pain.

The Feldenkrais Method® was developed by Moshe Feldenkrais, a physicist and martial arts practitioner. Feldenkrais developed his method while rehabilitating a knee injury. He studied anatomy and the science of movement in order to help himself learn to move without pain. Feldenkrais believed the key to pain-free movement was in better organization of movement patterns. This was accomplished through awareness of the body. He developed an active approach to instruct others in movement and a hands-on approach to work on releasing tension. He began teaching his method in the 1970s.

Awareness Through Movement® sessions are taught to groups of people. Students wear loose, comfortable clothing and are led through a series of slow, mindful exercises. While performing the exercises the students are invited to visualize and encouraged to sense the way they move. This helps them to coordinate their movements. An Awareness Through Movement® class can last 3–60 minutes. Functional Integration® sessions are private hands-on treatments that are performed with the client lying on a massage table wearing loose, comfortable clothing. Prior to the session, the practitioner interviews the client about his goals and needs. The practitioner creates a session that is tailored for the client. Gentle touch and passive movements are used to release tension and teach the client to move fluidly.

There is little research on benefits and applications for Feldenkrais.® Some practitioners report success in using Functional Integration® for individuals with ASD. The gentle touch and passive movements may be useful to improve proprioceptive awareness. Participating in Awareness Through Movement® classes may be challenging for individuals with ASD who have difficulty navigating a classroom setting. However, the emphasis on self-awareness and active movement may help to increase sensory awareness and improve coordination.

HELLERWORK

Hellerwork is a blend of movement education and connective tissue bodywork. It is based on techniques of Structural Integration and the belief that attitudes and emotions have profound influences on tension in the body. By encouraging understanding of the relationship between the mind and areas of tension in the body, a Hellerwork practitioner helps to restore freedom in movement.

Hellerwork, also called Hellerwork Structural Integration, was created in the 1970s by Joseph Heller. Heller was an engineer who developed an interest in bodywork and studied Structural Integration with Ida Rolf. Heller expanded on Rolf's ideas to create a body-mind therapy. He believed that pain and muscle imbalances could be corrected through a combination of massage, teaching people to be aware of their movement patterns, and helping people to understand how their muscles and posture are affected by their reaction to stress. Heller integrated aspects of Gestalt therapy to help clients understand the relationship between their mind and body. He believed that three components (massage, movement education, and awareness) would be more successful than a single approach to produce lasting benefits.

A standard Hellerwork approach consists of eleven 90-minute sessions. Prior to the session, the practitioner interviews the client and observes the client's posture and movements. For the bodywork, the client is partly clothed and lies on a massage table. Each session focuses on a specific area of the body and has a theme related to different stages of life or emotions. For example, the first few sessions in the series are related to early years of life. As the practitioner works to release tension, he or she engages in a dialogue with the client. The purpose of this dialogue is to help the client understand how specific areas of tension are related to long-held habits and beliefs. The sessions aim to create awareness of the emotional causes of tension and to let go of the emotions along with the release of tension in connective tissues.

There is no research on the benefits of Hellerwork for a typical population or for individuals with ASD. The connective tissue massage used in Hellerwork may be helpful to release tight muscles and fascia. For individuals with ASD who are non-verbal, the dialogue of Hellerwork poses a challenge. The aim of this style of bodywork is to relate psychological traits and emotions to physical tension. The effectiveness of this approach depends on the ability of the practitioner and client to communicate on a touch-based and verbal level. If a practitioner is willing and able to adapt the style to fit the needs of the client, the massage may increase physical awareness.

TRAGER® APPROACH

The Trager® Approach is a style of bodywork that uses rhythmic rocking movements and range of motion exercises to release tension and restore free movement. Also called Trager® Work or Trager® Psychophysical Integration, it was developed by Milton Trager, a physician, who intuitively created his own approach to bodywork. In response to his own physical limitations, Trager began to develop his work. After becoming a medical doctor, Trager began teaching his approach in the 1970s. He believed that deeply held emotions were related to physical tension and illnesses. By learning to move effortlessly and freely, a client could relieve stress and pain and improve their state of mind. Trager believed that his clients were students rather than patients. His work aimed to teach them how to move rather than attempt to cure a problem.

The passive and active movements used in Trager® are not a rigid system. Rather the techniques incorporate principles of the anatomy and physiology of movement, with special emphasis on reflexes. Different types of movements are used to stimulate reflexes and improve the coordination of muscles in movement. Trager includes passive table work that resembles massage and active movement instruction called Mentastics.® The passive rocking movements and joint range of motion used in the Trager® table work are intended to feel good and help the client experience joy in movement. Trager® practitioners focus on each individual client and choose techniques that they believe will help the particular area of the body move in a lighter and freer manner.

The movements used in Trager® are gentle, not forced. The goal of Trager® table work, where the client is lightly clothed and lying on a massage table, is to increase the client's awareness of the muscles and joints and introduce free movement. A Trager® session usually lasts 60–90 minutes and includes table work as well as active movement. Mentastics,® the active part of Trager,® teaches clients to move freely on their own. This requires mindfulness or awareness of the body-mind connection in movement. During the active part of the session, clients are guided in movements to learn how they can create the same free and light feeling they received on the table. Movements used in Mentastics® are taught so that the client can practice in between sessions.

Research on the Trager® Approach indicates that it can be beneficial in improving movement and relieving pain. There is no research on using the Trager® Approach for individuals with ASD. The passive Trager® table work may be useful in increasing sensory awareness and releasing tight fascia. The rhythmic shaking and jostling movements may be helpful with stress reduction and improving sleep. The movement education in Mentastics® may be challenging for individuals with ASD who have limited verbal skills or difficulty with attention. However, teaching a few gentle movements could be useful as a self-regulating tool to reduce outbursts related to anger or frustration.

ALEXANDER TECHNIQUE

Alexander Technique is movement education that teaches clients to understand and correct movement habits. Practitioners teach clients about using the proper balance, support, and effort to sit, stand, and move without tension. The foundation of Alexander Technique relies on bringing awareness to unnecessary tension in habitual movements. By learning to release tension a client can be guided to relearn how to move in an efficient way. The centerpiece of Alexander Technique is the mind-body connection.

Alexander Technique was developed by F. Matthais Alexander, an actor and voice teacher. Through his work and teaching, Alexander noticed a connection between the mind and physical tension in the body. He used breathing exercises and awareness training to release physical tension. This benefited his students on a psychological and emotional level. Alexander began teaching his technique in the 1890s and published his first book on the subject in 1910. Alexander Technique has been used extensively by performing artists to alleviate tension associated with singing, acting, and playing musical instruments.

Alexander Technique can be taught in private sessions or in small group classes. The clients wear loose comfortable clothing for sessions that usually last one hour. The practitioner observes the client's posture and how the client moves. Then using words, imagery, and touch, the practitioner guides the client to stand, sit, or move without unnecessary tension. The touch used in Alexander Technique is very gentle. The increased proprioceptive awareness in Alexander Technique is based on the client being aware of movement habits and corrected movement patterns.

There is a limited amount of research on Alexander Technique that suggests it can be helpful in reducing musculoskeletal pain and correcting muscle imbalances. Alexander Technique does not involve manipulation or stimulation like other forms of bodywork. While it is a body-mind approach that increases kinesthetic awareness, the success of a standard treatment relies on the client being able to respond to cues from the practitioner. This may be difficult for an individual with ASD who is hypo-sensitive to touch or has low physiological arousal. For those who are hyper-sensitive to touch and movement, Alexander Technique may be helpful in teaching them to understand and respond appropriately to physical sensations and movement.

PART 3

TRYING MASSAGE FOR YOUR CHILD

10 Choosing a Style of Massage

A parent or caregiver who is thinking about introducing their child to therapeutic massage and bodywork should start with this book. Read through the styles described in Chapters 7, 8, and 9. Parents should have a general understanding of the variety of options available. It is likely that something about one or more approaches will seem interesting, based on the child's sensory needs. Parents may also want to talk to friends and colleagues who get massages to find out what they like about different styles and how they enjoy the experience. A client's description can be a powerful testimonial.

Words give only a partial sense of the experience of massage. If possible, parents should experiment by receiving different styles of massage. This should be done with a purpose in mind: sensory activity and tactile training for a child. If a series of massages is not financially feasible, it is usually possible to schedule short samples of multiple styles from an eclectic practitioner. This will give the parent or caregiver an idea of what the client will experience. It is important to remember that massage is a personal, sensory experience. A parent may prefer light pressure and techniques, which may be irritating or uninteresting to a hypo-sensitive child. While the experience may be enjoyable for the parent, try to see it through the eyes of your child. The goal in finding a style and a practitioner is to benefit the child.

After one or more styles have been identified and a practitioner is located, the success of massage treatment depends on how massage benefits the client. Similar to other therapies for ASD, the practitioner will need to develop a rapport with the client and experiment with approaches. The client should be asked and observed for feedback by the practitioner and the caregiver. Once a massage treatment and sequence is established, the client should receive the treatment on a regularly scheduled basis. This may involve weekly scheduled massage treatments. More likely it will involve the practitioner teaching the parent how to massage the child so that the massages can be performed on a more regular basis. Occasional check-ins with the massage practitioner can help maintain consistency in treatment and allow time to observe changes that occur as a result of the massage. This approach, often used in research, usually makes massage more accessible.

FINDING A PRACTITIONER

There are many massage practitioners with a variety of training. According to the U.S. Department of Labor, massage therapists may specialize in eighty different recognized styles of massage. That offers many options for the client with ASD.

It is important to select a practitioner who is compassionate, experienced with practicing massage, and flexible in adapting massage treatment. Ideally a practitioner should be conveniently located and offer affordable rates. The massage and bodywork professional should take time for a phone consultation and be willing to answer questions. Practitioners who are experienced in working with children and clients with special needs will understand that extra time and effort are important. Taking time to play and laugh with the client may be necessary in order to develop a rapport.

Many massage therapists are self-employed or work part-time. A good place to start looking for a massage professional is to ask for recommendations or referrals. Ask other members of the ASD therapy team or friends and colleagues who get massages. Some massage schools or massage continuing education providers have alumni directories. There are many different regional and national associations with searchable directories that can be accessed on the Internet. Typing the massage-style words into an Internet browser tool usually yields results to use as a starting point. When a practitioner is located, parents should interview them about their qualifications, skills, training, and experience. It is important to remember that all professional practitioners should comply with local laws for licensure or certification.

Be wary of any practitioner who claims they can cure ASD using massage or bodywork. Massage is another tool, just like sensory integration work, exercise, and fine-motor skill activities. Rarely does a basic, scripted massage protocol benefit every client. Massage almost always needs to be adapted and adjusted in some way to best meet individual client needs. That means that the pace, rhythm, amount of pressure, or sequence may be individualized. While there may be similarities in different therapeutic approaches, few successful ASD therapies use a cookie-cutter formula. Any massage practitioner should be willing to teach the parent or caregiver touch strategies and massage techniques. Most professional massage practitioners are aware of the research that substantiates the benefits of teaching parents to massage their children. Findings have consistently noted benefits for the child and for the parent who is given a positive tool to help their child.

Not every massage and bodywork professional will necessarily have the skills or patience to work with a client who has special needs. Unlike many other allied health professionals, most massage therapists are trained to work with reasonably healthy adults. They may be unaccustomed to working with children or with a client who has difficulty communicating. It is important to keep in mind that a massage practitioner who declines to work with an individual with ASD is not unprofessional. Rather, they may lack adequate training or experience with children. They may be able to refer you to other, qualified practitioners.

Some conventional healthcare professionals are enthusiastic about massage. In particular, some nurses use massage techniques as part of nursing practice. They may give a patient a back rub or foot massage after a bath. Pediatric nurses are sometimes trained to massage premature infants to encourage weight gain. This enthusiasm and practice give credibility to the use of massage techniques, but the training for nurses and other healthcare professionals in massage is far less than training required for professional massage practitioners. Therefore, someone trained to teach general infant massage to new parents will not generally have the same skills, techniques, or creativity as a massage professional who is trained and experienced in massage.

LAWS REGULATING MASSAGE

The legal regulation of massage is inconsistent around the world. In many countries it is regulated on a regional basis, while in others it is not regulated at all. Where massage laws are in effect, regulation may cover practitioners, establishments, or both. That means that the massage practitioner and the facility where they practice massage must meet minimum professional standards. Massage professionals may practice in health clubs, day spas, wellness centers, rehabilitation settings, or even at shopping malls or airport kiosks, and out of the home. The setting does not determine what type of massage is practiced. Regulation of the settings usually is concerned with cleanliness, hygiene, and business licenses.

The purpose of regulating massage is to protect the public. Regulation helps that by requiring massage practitioners to meet a minimum training standard. This section is concerned with the certification and licensing of practitioners.

In the United States, Canada, and the United Kingdom, massage is not nationally regulated. Some massage practitioners are licensed at the state or province level. In states or provinces that lack licenses, massage practitioners may be licensed by the county or city. Sometimes massage is not regulated at all. In areas where massage practice is regulated, education and curriculum requirements are in place that serve as minimum standards for certification or licensure. In all areas, education standards require study of human anatomy, physiology, training in massage techniques and ethics, as well as the supervised practice of massage. Some areas require additional training in the science of movement (kinesiology), spa therapies, multiple styles of massage, and the use of hot and cold therapies (hydrotherapy).

In the United States, the education requirements range from 250 to 1000 hours of training. Throughout most of the United States, 500 hours of massage training is required.

Canadian regulations range from 2200 to 3000 hours of training. Voluntary registration is used for massage therapists in the United Kingdom with various levels of training. Education and training in massage requires classroom time in the presence of an instructor. For massage techniques and practicum (supervised practice of massage) the instructor must be an experienced, licensed or certified massage therapist. Science courses such as anatomy and physiology, kinesiology, or stretching are sometimes taught by other healthcare professionals like chiropractors, medical doctors, or nurses.

Massage training programs can be found in private schools, vocational schools, and academically accredited colleges. The massage student may earn a certificate, diploma, or academic degree depending on the accreditation of the school. Once a student completes a training program, the massage professional may be registered as required by regulation. In locations that register massage professionals, proof of completion of an approved curriculum is required to register. Some areas require an examination for massage license or certification. Successful completion of the examination is required for professional licensure or certification to practice massage.

Some areas require massage professionals to complete professional continuing education courses. These courses usually cover advanced topics, different techniques or styles of massage, or timely topics such as research updates. Certification or certification of completion is given to verify that these professional education courses are finished. It is important to note that specialty certifications are not required for massage professionals to practice different styles of massage. Once professionals meet license or certification requirements for their area, they are free to practice any style of massage.

The regulation for bodywork adds some confusion. Styles that do not involve manipulation or stroking of the skin or muscles are not considered massage in many areas and therefore are not subject to the same licensing or certification laws as massage. For example, yoga teachers, Pilates trainers, and personal trainers may stretch clients and educate them about movement but they are not licensed to massage. That means that these individuals may not practice massage, but they may engage in hands-on work that is customary to their occupation. Practitioners of bodywork styles like Alexander Technique and Feldenkrais® are not always subject to massage regulation because these styles emphasize active movement rather than touch-based therapies. Interpretation of regulations is sometimes confusing to the practitioners who may wish to add massage to their practice. Any person who has a question about the credentials of a practitioner can contact the state or province office that oversees regulation of massage. This is important for parents to remember, especially since laws are in place to protect clients from potential harm.

In addition to the marginalization of massage as an alternative therapy, another factor has influenced the limited use of professional massage for ASD. That involves the substantial variety that exists within the massage profession. Different titles are used to refer to a person who performs massage including: massage practitioner, massage therapist, masseuse, masseur, massotherapist, or myotherapist. Massage professionals work in different settings such as beauty spas, chiropractic offices, sports medicine facilities, or fitness centers. Titles and locations do not consistently indicate what type of massage is performed or techniques used. In other words, a person could receive an orthopedic massage at a day spa or a relaxation massage at a rehabilitation center. One would expect the relaxation massage to occur at a day spa and the orthopedic massage to occur at a rehabilitation center. When potential clients understand that the technique or style is not dependent on the setting, it is easier to understand that massage is a very flexible treatment. The names, terminology, and setting do not disguise the fact that the treatment is massage.

The scope of practice for massage professionals is an important consideration for parents and caregivers. In areas where massage is regulated by law, the practice is limited to massage therapists or other professionals who are trained and licensed to use massage techniques. Some legislation specifically recognizes that the use of some massage techniques is appropriate within the professional scope of athletic trainers, physical therapists, chiropractors, certain healthcare providers, and even barbers. This means that professionals like chiropractors and physical therapists may perform massage or stretch patients as part of treatments. Nurses may be able to give foot or back rubs within the context of nursing care. Occupational therapists may use stretching or rubbing techniques in sensory therapy. Personal trainers and other fitness professionals may stretch clients. Barbers and hair stylists can also give a neck massage in a manner that is customary to their occupational setting. However, the only professional that is legally licensed to give a full session is a certified, licensed, or registered massage practitioner. This is an important distinction for parents who are seeking massage.

A massage practitioner can teach a parent or caregiver to massage their child or other individual under their care. However, that does not mean that the parent can massage other people or other children. This is similar to a parent who is taught to administer a medication to a child. Learning how to give a shot or change a dressing on a wound does not qualify the parent to perform medical care on others. Many people have enthusiasm for massage and bodywork, but law and regulations exist to protect the public from harm. The training required by law is generally believed to be a minimum standard to promote safe practice. Most practitioners would agree that experience and further training enhance their skills and abilities.

Another consideration about regulation of massage is the scope of massage practice. Massage practitioners may massage, press, rub, knead, stretch, or use other soft-tissue techniques. They may teach clients stretching or self-massage, but they may not teach fitness or prescribe exercise unless they are trained and certified in fitness or exercise. Massage practitioners are not legally qualified to give nutritional advice, prescribe herbs, vitamins, or medications. Apart from the dialogue used in some forms of bodywork, massage professionals are also not permitted to provide psychotherapy, mental health counseling, or family therapy. Massage therapists do not diagnose illness or disease. When a client has symptoms or signs of a disorder, the massage therapist will conduct an assessment and develop a treatment plan tailored to meet the needs of the client. This is possible because massage practitioners are trained to understand fundamentals of pathological conditions. A massage professional can and should refer a client to a licensed medical care provider in order to have a suspected medical condition accurately diagnosed. A prescription is not required to receive a massage, but a physician may refer patients to massage practitioners or recommend massage. Since physicians and nurse practitioners are not trained in massage techniques, generally such a referral is the use of massage to treat signs or symptoms of a medical condition. The choice of techniques is up to the massage practitioner.

HEALTH INSURANCE REIMBURSEMENT

As of this writing, massage is not widely covered by health insurance in the United States. Some insurers in Canada and the United Kingdom will reportedly cover massage. There are insurance companies that reimburse patients for massage that is prescribed by a physician. Workers compensation insurance policies sometimes cover payment for massage that is related to a workplace injury. A few insurance companies provide lists of massage practitioners as a service to their insured. However, it is important to note that such a list is usually just a referral method. The treatment is not necessarily a covered benefit that is reimbursed by the insurance company. Parents should contact their child's insurance provider to understand possible coverage for massage. If a referral is accepted, the child's pediatrician or physician should be consulted to obtain a referral. Parents can also ask individual massage practitioners about their relationships with insurance companies.

When massage is not generally covered by insurance, massage treatments must be paid at time of service. There are many possibilities to help make massage more affordable. Some practitioners and facilities offer package discounts when sessions are purchased in a series. Since introducing a child to massage is a gradual process, parents could split a scheduled massage session with their child. Several children with ASD could be grouped together into a single appointment timeslot.

More research that substantiates the benefits of massage to treat signs and symptoms of illnesses and diseases is necessary if insurance companies will be expected to cover massage treatments. Until that time, the lack of insurance reimbursement will likely remain a barrier for parents who may pay out of pocket for other services for their child. Parents should contact a massage practitioner to inquire about possibilities to make massage accessible and affordable. The possibility of teaching parents how to massage may help overcome the insurance barrier.

CONTRAINDICATIONS AND PRECAUTIONS

In general, therapeutic massage and bodywork can be performed on almost anyone. However, there are some conditions that are not appropriate for massage (contraindicated) or for which massage treatment should be modified (precaution). Massage and bodywork are contraindicated when the client or the practitioner has an infectious disease. This includes skin conditions (rashes, fungal infections), respiratory diseases (influenza, common cold), digestive disorders (virus or bacterial infection), or other contagious conditions. In such situations massage should not be performed because of the risk of passing along the contagious condition. Massage is also contraindicated if the client is under the influence of alcohol, recreational drugs, or mind-altering substances.

There are several situations where precautions are necessary for massage. If the client has inflammation, history of heart disease, a blood pressure disorder, or is pregnant, massage treatment should be modified. Certain disorders such as hemophilia, osteoporosis, or history of joint dislocation require precautions so the client is not injured during massage treatment. Because of the risk of infection, skin with open wounds should not be massaged. Precautions are also important if the client is taking medications for pain relief or to decrease blood clotting.

Massage is also not recommended if the client will not tolerate touch. It is important to remember that introducing a child with ASD to massage may take several attempts. These attempts often require experimentation with massage and bodywork styles or appointments with different practitioners. The child should always be informed about the massage and given the opportunity to ask questions if possible. When that is not feasible, massage should be gradually introduced. Massage should make the client feel better, rather than worse.

Because massage is a passive treatment, precautions are important for an individual with ASD. Matching the massage treatment to the child's needs takes time and experimentation. The child and the parents should be informed about the treatment and given the opportunity to ask questions. A child who is unable to give verbal consent should be observed for positive and negative feedback in his or her behavior and body language.

11
Massage for Children

SPECIAL CONSIDERATIONS

Professional massage therapists and bodyworkers are trained to work with clients of all ages. Many practitioners who work in health clubs, chiropractic offices, with athletic teams, or at spas work only with adults. Working with children takes a different type of patience and creativity. Special certifications and supplemental training beyond licensure or certification are not necessary to work with children or an individual who has special needs. What is important is that the needs of the client are taken into consideration in the design of the massage treatment. When massaging a child, the practitioner should help the child to understand what will happen during massage, obtain consent, introduce the child to the treatment, and solicit feedback. Sometimes playing can help to establish a rapport.

PREPARING THE CHILD FOR MASSAGE

Massage is a wonderful therapy, but many people have questions about massage before receiving a treatment. Prior to scheduling a massage, the practitioner should be willing to provide information on the styles and techniques that they use, describe a basic treatment, and answer questions. This will help the parents and the child know what to expect from massage. For a child with ASD, the practitioner should also be prepared to evaluate and alter the treatment as necessary. Often this is in response to observations during the first few treatments. The parent or caregiver is the best expert in observing their child's behavior. Working with the practitioner will provide information and help with the success of massage treatment.

Since a massage for an individual with ASD should be tailored to meet the client's sensory needs, the practitioner should conduct a thorough interview. In addition to a confidential health history and energy evaluation (if applicable), the practitioner may ask questions about the child's self-stimulating behaviors, motor skills, and any displays of touch aversion. The practitioner should ask about successes and challenges in sensory therapy and tactile training. The practitioner should also have the opportunity to observe the child prior to massage. Watching a child play or move can help the practitioner understand the child in a similar way to a massage practitioner who watches an athlete or dancer perform, examines a client working at a desk, or observes a musician play an instrument. Such observations can be useful in understanding how movement or activity relates to posture, alignment, or muscle or fascia injuries. For a client with ASD, observation can provide information about their motor skills and sensory preferences. All of this information provides clues to the types of massage techniques that the child may be willing to receive. Since introducing the child to massage will be an evolving process, the pre-massage assessment will help the practitioner begin to make choices about developing a massage sequence.

INFORMATION AND CONSENT

For each and every massage client, understanding what to expect and consenting to receive massage is important. In medical care this is called *informed consent*. The client should be informed about what will happen in the treatment session, how long it will take, whether there are expected risks or anticipated benefits, and if there are alternative treatments or techniques that may produce a similar result. If the client is a child (usually that means anyone under age 18), a parent or guardian may be required to sign a consent form for the child to receive a massage treatment.

All children—regardless of age or verbal skills—should be informed about the massage and given the opportunity to consent. When a client has limited communication skills, obtaining consent can sometimes be a difficult process. Interviewing a parent about the child's behaviors and communication techniques can help the practitioner read and understand the child's behavioral cues. For example, shaking the head side-to-side could mean "no" or it could be a form of visual or vestibular stimulating behavior. Understanding the difference is important. For non-verbal children, consent can be described using sign language, pictures, or words. Regardless of a child's verbal ability, the child should be informed about the massage. Many children need to be coaxed into trying new things, and a child with ASD is no exception. Massage should be introduced gently in a fun and relaxing way. The practitioner will need to experiment with techniques, but a child should not be forced into anything. A few sessions may be needed to help the child understand what massage is about. Practice and research findings indicate that children are excited to receive massage once they know what to expect from a treatment.[37]

Every client, regardless of their age, should be educated about their rights to privacy: who can touch them and where on their body it is appropriate to touch. It is never appropriate to expose or massage genitals. Although many massage types are typically performed without clothing on adults, the client is covered with a sheet or towel. This can be problematic for children, who are often active during massage. They should remain clothed to protect their modesty. A T-shirt or tank top and shorts can be worn during massage. Most massage and bodywork styles can be adapted easily for this type of clothing. Sometimes bathing suits are recommended for children, but for a special needs child it is probably not a good choice for an outfit. A child who is dressed for swimming may be more interested in going to the pool than receiving a massage. Pajamas are associated with bedtime, so that is also not a good clothing choice. What is important is that the clothing is comfortable and the child is not exposed in an uncomfortable manner.

During the first few massage sessions, a parent or caregiver should be present. This is especially important for small children, even though the presence of a parent may be distracting for the child. When the parent and child are comfortable, the parent can leave the room but should remain nearby. Having the parent sit quietly outside the door or around a corner out of sight is a good solution. This helps the parent feel comfortable while enabling the child to relax and receive massage.

INTRODUCING THE CHILD TO MASSAGE

The child needs time to become familiar with the massage therapist, the massage setting, and receiving touch. For children with ASD who are used to traveling for therapy sessions, a visit to a massage practitioner's office may be fun and appropriate. However, if the child is used to participating in therapy at home, then a house call will help the child be comfortable.

A professional massage office should be child-friendly but not overwhelming. Most massage rooms are dark with candles and soothing music. When the massage room is dimly lit, it may be difficult for the child to understand or feel comfortable. Often a dark room means bedtime—something many children try to avoid—so that can make them anxious. From a safety perspective, candlelight is not a good idea. A comfortable room with indirect or low-level lighting will help most children relax. The room should have an unobtrusive place for a parent to sit.

A home-based massage setting usually needs to be creatively configured. For a child who has a dedicated sensory or therapy space, massage can take place in that area of the house. The space should have ample room for the practitioner and the child. It should also be free of breakable objects or furniture with sharp corners. Often young children move around and wiggle during the massage. That can be dangerous if a child is massaged on a bed or a couch. Sometimes substantial effort is needed to keep them from falling, which can take away from the massage. The child could be massaged on the floor lying on a mat or pillows. This keeps the child in a safe position so they cannot fall and will have room to wiggle around.

Small children can be easily held and massaged by the practitioner or by parents during a session. Not only can this help the massage environment be safe, but also it can help the child feel comfortable and nurtured (see Figure 11.1). Young children often need some type of distraction. Letting children play with a favorite toy can help them feel comfortable. Massage therapists who work with children often keep a small number of toys on hand like small balls, plastic massage tools, soft towels, or fleece blankets which can easily be cleaned between sessions.

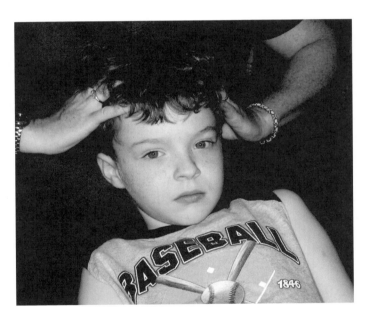

Figure 11.1 Scalp massage

While receiving massage, young children need help focusing. The massage therapist can sing, tell stories, or play counting or word games. This is different than the usual protocol followed when massaging an adult, although adults sometimes talk while being massaged. Playing videos is not a good idea for a child with sensory issues. They may get distracted and become involved in the visual or auditory stimulus making them less open to receive and understand touch. Limiting distracting sights and sounds can help the child focus on their own physical awareness. For children who have had success with music therapy, soft music with a rhythmic, moderately slow beat can help the child to relax. Drumming soundtracks, Baroque classical music, or other music without words with a predictable cadence around 60 beats per minute are usually good choices. Aromatherapy diffused in the massage room or added to lotion or oil may also help the child relax. Research has not found substantial evidence that aromatherapy massage is beneficial in helping children with ASD to sleep, but it may help them relax.[38,39] It is important to remember that too many different stimuli—sights, sounds, smells, and touch—can take away the focus on receiving touch.

It is not unusual for a child with ASD to vocalize, giggle, or even cry during the massage. Children who vocalize during massage may actually be trying to feel the sound of their own voice or the movement of their tongue and lips. Sometimes they do not have words to say that they are happy. Infants and young children frequently cry when they are first massaged. The crying usually contrasts with their body language. For example, children will often be physically relaxed during the massage and exhibit movements that are receptive to touch while simultaneously crying or vocalizing. Generally when children cry because they are upset, their body is tense and rigid. This somatic difference during massage may be difficult for parents to understand at first. But, children who cry or fuss during their first few ten-minute massages will usually cry or fuss only at the beginning after they receive a few massages. Once children know what to expect, they will demonstrate enjoyment and may even ask for massage.[40]

Children should be relaxed and well rested when they receive massage. It is not a good idea to schedule massage immediately after a stimulating activity or soon after eating. To introduce a child to massage, the practitioner may split a session between the child and the parent. Giving the child the opportunity to observe a massage will make it more familiar. Initially, massage sessions may need to be short (even ten minutes) especially for young children. Older children may be able to begin with longer sessions (twenty minutes). The length of the session can increase over time as the child becomes more comfortable and knows what to expect.

GROWTH AND DEVELOPMENT

Throughout the phases of growth and development, there are special considerations for massage. From infants to older adults, the practitioner must consider physical and behavioral needs of each client. The muscles and joints in children are flexible compared to adults. Pressure should be modified to take this into account. Even though they are flexible, children should never be over stretched. Some of the bones (for example the skull) fuse during development and others do not reach full growth until adolescence. During the growing years, bone density is not fully established. Thus, care should be taken when massaging certain areas.

Children are more sensitive to changes in temperature than adults. Young children are also not able to sweat effectively, so the massage area should not be too warm, which may make the child uncomfortable. Unlike most adults, children need to be encouraged to relax. During the massage, the practitioner observes the child for signs of relaxation. As a person relaxes, the heart rate and breathing rate become slower. A child's heart rate and breathing (respiratory) rate are faster than that of an adult but will still slow down as the child relaxes.

Appropriate response to stimuli is something that typical children learn with time and experience. There will be signals during the massage that a child is responsive to massage. More important for a child with ASD is observation of positive or negative changes after massage. Parents should note changes in tactile behaviors, verbal communication, self-stimulating activities, and even diet. Some children are more willing to eat different foods after receiving massage.

LEARNING MASSAGE FOR PARENTS AND CAREGIVERS

Making massage part of an ASD individual's therapy routine is important so that they learn how to receive and respond to touch. Daily visits to a massage therapist are not usually possible or feasible. Try to find a massage therapist who is willing to combine regular professional massage appointments with instruction on how the parent can massage the child on a regular basis. The practitioner can train the parent to perform simple massage sequences. It is important for the parent to learn to use the right amount of pressure and pacing. Not only can this help the child's progress, but also it can help add something to the "tool kit" that nearly every parent of a child with ASD needs. Regular check-ins with the massage therapist can help parents to adapt their massage as the child develops.

Even a busy parent has the opportunity to massage a child on a regular basis. A short massage routine performed a few days each week can become part of the home therapy routine for a child with ASD. Research protocols that have evaluated the benefits of massage for children with ASD use both practitioners and parents to give massage. This has been found to benefit both the child and the parents.[41–46]

A parent or caregiver for an individual with ASD should use any opportunity for touch as a tactile learning experience. This includes daily hygiene. Bath time can be quite traumatic for some children. Even a few massage techniques can help a bath-resisting child to relax and feel good. Massaging the child's head while shampooing or selecting a washcloth or bath sponge of the right texture can turn bath time into a therapeutic adventure. Compression of the arm and leg muscles can be easily combined into toweling-off after a bath.

Application of sunscreen or lotion can also be challenging, but offers another massage opportunity. Working with a massage therapist to understand a child's preference for massage strokes can help parents learn how to use the right touch techniques and even a predictable sequence. That can help reduce tantrums and frustration that may result from touch that is perceived as irritating or unpleasant.

A gentle massage using slow strokes can help relax a child at bedtime. The pressure should be adjusted so that it is light enough—or deep enough—to meet the child's sensory needs. But a word of caution! If parents choose to massage their child—and they only do so at bedtime—the child may equate massage with going to sleep. That child may grow to dislike massage because it means bedtime is near.

A professional practitioner can and should help a parent or caregiver to learn how to touch and massage the child in a manner that will be well received. The goal of the touch and massage is to increase touch receptiveness, which can open a door to other types of communication. Teaching the parent or caregiver does not license them to massage other adults or children. That is an important legal distinction.

COORDINATING MASSAGE WITH THE THERAPY TEAM

There is a variety of fantastic benefits of massage and bodywork. Regardless of the style, massage is a very useful complementary therapy for ASD. Even a small amount of massage can be helpful in reducing self-stimulating behaviors and encouraging receptiveness to touch. Ideally, massage is a complementary therapy activity. Massage and other sensory therapies can help to provide stimulus, release muscle contractures, balance energy, and improve receptivity to touch. Massage and bodywork should not attempt to replace sensory integration, speech, or occupational therapy. Parents and caregivers should keep a treatment log of massage and other sensory activities. This can help monitor progress and changes over time.

Massage treatments, whether professionally administered or given by a parent or caregiver, should be scheduled around other therapy activities. Scheduling, organization, and consistency are important for many individuals with ASD. Making a commitment to trying massage for a period of time is usually necessary to observe positive changes. Many parents of children with an ASD are willing to try multiple interventions. That can sometimes be confusing for the child. It also can be difficult to document the benefits of individual therapies. Introducing massage as a complementary therapy should be done carefully to help the child understand what is going on and to aid the parent in monitoring positive changes for their child.

Healthcare information, including details about massage treatment, is confidential. This information should not be shared with other people, including health and medical care practitioners, by anyone other than the client (or parent) without consent. Yet, it is important to inform members of the client's therapy team that the client is receiving massage.

Letting the others know can help them to understand sensory and behavioral changes that they might observe. The massage professional may also be able to educate the parent on certain techniques that work well—or not. That can be useful in helping the occupational therapist or physical therapist better understand how to meet the client's needs.

Since massage is an alternative therapy, many conventional medical practitioners are not aware of what massage is or how it works. Unfortunately that means the parents may encounter resistance from other healthcare providers when they opt to try massage. What is important to remember is that massage is a touch-based therapy that is truly an extension of other sensory activities like stretching and brushing. The choice to try massage lies with the parents and the client. There is little evidence to suggest that massage is harmful for ASD. Massage is enjoyable. Nearly anyone can learn to enjoy massage when their preferences for being touched are considered in the massage treatment.

Some conventional medical practitioners may be enthusiastic about a single massage style based on their own familiarity or experience. They may wish to experiment with techniques on the child. In general, that is not a good idea. A more eclectic or flexible approach is often needed to meet the sensory needs for an individual with ASD. The only person well trained enough to experiment with giving massage is a trained and qualified massage practitioner.

REFERENCES

1. Beider, S. and C.A. Moyer, "Randomized controlled trials of pediatric massage: a review." *Evidence-Based Complementary and Alternative Medicine,* 2007. **4**(1): 23–34.

2. Field, T., "Massage therapy for infants and children." *Journal of Developmental and Behavioral Pediatrics,* 1995. **16**(2): 105–111.

3. Field, T., *Massage therapy research.* 2006, Edinburgh: Churchill Livingstone.

4. Escalona, A., T. Field, R. Singer-Strunch, C. Cullen, and K. Hartshorn, "Brief report: improvements in the behavior of children with autism following massage therapy." *Journal of Autism and Developmental Disorders,* 2001. **31**(5): 513–516.

5. Field, T., D. Lasko, P. Mundy, T. Henteleff, *et al.,* "Brief report: autistic children's attentiveness and responsivity improve after touch therapy." *Journal of Autism and Developmental Disorders,* 1997. **27**(3): 333–338.

6. Sapolsky, R.M., *Why zebras don't get ulcers: an updated guide to stress, stress-related diseases, and coping.* 1998, New York: W.H. Freeman.

7. Burdea, G. and P. Coiffet, *Virtual reality technology,* 2nd edn. 2003, Hoboken, NJ: Wiley-IEEE Press.

8.   Melzack, R. and P.D. Wall, "Pain mechanisms: a new theory." *Science,* 1965. **150**(699): 971–979.

9.   Melzack, R., "Pain and the neuromatrix in the brain." *Journal of Dental Education,* 2001. **65**(12): 1378–1382.

10. Burdea, G. and P. Coiffet, *Virtual reality technology,* 2nd edn. 2003, Hoboken, NJ: Wiley-IEEE Press.

11. Gallace, A. and C. Spence, "The science of interpersonal touch: an overview." *Neuroscience and Biobehavioral Reviews,* 2010. **34**(2): 246–259.

12. Fisher, J.D., M. Rytting, and R. Heslin, "Hands touching hands: affective and evaluative effects of an interpersonal touch." *Sociometry,* 1976. **39**(4): 416–421.

13. Coleman, M., ed. *The neurology of autism.* 2005, New York: Oxford University Press.

14. Plaisted, K., J. Swettenham, and L. Rees, "Children with autism show local precedence in a divided attention task and global precedence in a selective attention task." *Journal of Child Psychology and Psychiatry,* 1999. **40**(5): 733–742.

15. Remington, A., J. Swettenham, R. Campbell, and M. Coleman, "Selective attention and perceptual load in autism spectrum disorder." *Psychological Science,* 2009. **20**(11): 1388–1393.

16. Barnett-Cowan, M. and L.R. Harris, "Perceived timing of vestibular stimulation relative to touch, light and sound." *Experimental Brain Research,* 2009. **198**(2–3): 221–231.

17. Moyer, C.A., J. Rounds, and J.W. Hannum, "A meta-analysis of massage therapy research." *Psychological Bulletin,* 2004. **130**(1): 3–18.

18. Escalona, A., T. Field, R. Singer-Strunch, C. Cullen, and K. Hartshorn, "Brief report: improvements in the behavior of children with autism following massage therapy." *Journal of Autism and Developmental Disorders,* 2001. **31**(5): 513–516.

19. Field, T., D. Lasko, P. Mundy, T. Henteleff, *et al.,* "Brief report: autistic children's attentiveness and responsivity improve after touch therapy." *Journal of Autism and Developmental Disorders,* 1997. **27**(3): 333–338.

20. Cullen-Powell, L.A., J.H. Barlow, and D. Cushway, "Exploring a massage intervention for parents and their children with autism: the implications for bonding and attachment." *Journal of Child Health Care,* 2005. **9**: 245–255.

21. Coleman, M., ed. *The neurology of autism.* 2005, New York: Oxford University Press.

22. Upledger, J.E. and J.D. Vredevoogd, *Craniosacral therapy*. 1983, Seattle, WA: Eastland Press.

23. Zhang, J., "A review of autism spectrum disorders (ASD) from a perspective of classical Chinese medicine (CCM)." *Journal of Traditional Chinese Medicine*, 2010. **30**(1): 53–59.

24. Silva, L.M., R. Ayres, and M. Schalock, "Outcomes of a pilot training program in a qigong massage intervention for young children with autism." *American Journal of Occupational Therapy*, 2008. **62**(5): 538–546.

25. Silva, L.M. and A. Cignolini, "A medical qigong methodology for early intervention in autism spectrum disorder: a case series." *American Journal of Chinese Medicine*, 2005. **33**(2): 315–327.

26. Silva, L.M., A. Cignolini, R. Warren, S. Budden, and A. Skowron-Gooch, "Improvement in sensory impairment and social interaction in young children with autism following treatment with an original Qigong massage methodology." *American Journal of Chinese Medicine*, 2007. **35**(3): 393–406.

27. Silva, L.M., M. Schalock, R. Ayres, C. Bunse, and S. Budden, "Qigong massage treatment for sensory and self-regulation problems in young children with autism: a randomized controlled trial." *American Journal of Occupational Therapy*, 2009. **63**(4): 423–432.

28. Chokevivat, V. and A. Chuthaputti, "The role of Thai traditional medicine in health promotion," in *Sixth Global Conference on Health Promotion*. 2005, Bangkok, Thailand: Department for the Development of Thai Traditional and Alternative Medicine, Ministry of Public Health.

29. Piravej, K., P. Tangtrongchitr, P. Chandarasiri, L. Paothong, and S. Sukprasong, "Effects of Thai traditional massage on autistic children's behavior." *Journal of Alternative and Complementary Medicine*, 2009. **15**(12): 1355–1361.

30. Ireland, M. and M. Olson, "Massage therapy and therapeutic touch in children: state of the science." *Alternative Therapies in Health and Medicine*, 2000. **6**(5): 54–63.

31. Kemper, K.J. and E.A. Kelly, "Treating children with therapeutic and healing touch." *Pediatric Annals*, 2004. **33**(4): 248–252.

32. Monroe, C.M., "The effects of therapeutic touch on pain." *Journal of Holistic Nursing*, 2009. **27**(2): 85–92.

33. Winstead-Fry, P. and J. Kijek, "An integrative review and meta-analysis of therapeutic touch research." *Alternative Therapies in Health and Medicine*, 1999. **5**(6): 58–67.

34. Vonder Hulls, D.S., L.K. Walker, and J.M. Powell, "Clinicians' perceptions of the benefits of aquatic therapy for young children with autism: a preliminary study." *Physical and Occupational Therapy in Pediatrics*, 2006. **26**(1–2): 13–22.

35. Getz, M., Y. Hutzler, and A. Vermeer, "Effects of aquatic interventions in children with neuromotor impairments: a systematic review of the literature." *Clinical Rehabilitation*, 2006. **20**(11): 927–936.

36. Johnson, C.C., "The benefits of physical activity for youth with developmental disabilities: a systematic review." *American Journal of Health Promotion*, 2009. **23**(3): 157–167.

37. Cullen-Powell, L.A., J.H. Barlow, and D. Cushway, "Exploring a massage intervention for parents and their children with autism: the implications for bonding and attachment." *Journal of Child Health Care*, 2005. **9**(4): 245–255.

38. Williams, T.I., "Evaluating effects of aromatherapy massage on sleep in children with autism: a pilot study." *Evidence-Based Complementary and Alternative Medicine*, 2006. **3**(3): 373–377.

39. Solomons, S., "Using aromatherapy massage to increase shared attention behaviours in children with autistic spectrum disorders and severe learning difficulties." *British Journal of Special Education*, 2005. **32**(3): 127–137.

40. Cullen, L.A., J.H. Barlow, and D. Cushway, "Positive touch, the implications for parents and their children with autism: an exploratory study." *Complementary Therapies in Clinical Practice*, 2005. **11**(3): 182–189.

41. Silva, L.M., R. Ayres, and M. Schalock, "Outcomes of a pilot training program in a qigong massage intervention for young children with autism." *American Journal of Occupational Therapy*, 2008. **62**(5): 538–546.

42. Williams, T.I., "Evaluating effects of aromatherapy massage on sleep in children with autism: a pilot study." *Evidence-Based Complementary and Alternative Medicine*, 2006. **3**(3): 373–377.

43. Solomons, S., "Using aromatherapy massage to increase shared attention behaviours in children with autistic spectrum disorders and severe learning difficulties." *British Journal of Special Education*, 2005. **32**(3): 127–137.

44. Cullen, L.A., J.H. Barlow, and D. Cushway, "Positive touch, the implications for parents and their children with autism: an exploratory study." *Complementary Therapies in Clinical Practice*, 2005. **11**(3): 182–189.

45. Cullen, L. and J. Barlow, "'Kiss, cuddle, squeeze': the experiences and meaning of touch among parents of children with autism attending a Touch Therapy Programme." *Journal of Child Health Care*, 2002. **6**(3): 171–181.

46. Escalona, A., T. Field, R. Singer-Strunch, C. Cullen, and K. Hartshorn, "Brief report: improvements in the behavior of children with autism following massage therapy." *Journal of Autism and Developmental Disorders*, 2001. **31**(5): 513–516.

USEFUL RESOURCES

American Massage Therapy Association
    www.amtamassage.org

American Organization for Bodywork Therapies of Asia
    www.aobta.org

American Reflexology Certification Board
    http://arcb.net/cms

Associated Bodywork & Massage Professionals
    www.abmp.com

Association of Holistic Biodynamic Massage Therapists
    www.ahbmt.org

Complementary and Natural Healthcare Council
    www.cnhc.org.uk

General Council for Massage Therapies
    www.gcmt.org.uk

International Register of Massage Therapists
    www.irmt.co.uk

Irish Massage Therapists Association
    www.massageireland.org

London and Counties Society of Physiologists
www.lcsp.uk.com

Massage Magazine
www.massagemag.com/Resources/massage-laws-legislation.php

Massage Therapists' Association of British Columbia
www.massagetherapy.bc.ca

Massage Therapy in Canada
www.massage.ca

Massage Therapy UK
www.massagetherapy.co.uk

National Association of Massage and Manipulative Therapists
www.nammt.co.uk

National Certification Board for Therapeutic Massage and Bodywork
www.ncbtmb.org

Scottish Massage Therapists Organisation
www.scotmass.co.uk

INDEX